GOOD HEALTH MAY BE AT HAND!

It may be as close as your garden, or even your kitchen cabinets. Effective, inexpensive—and unexpected—here is just a sampling of what healthful simple things may be within your reach at this very moment:

WITCH HAZEL—astringent, sedative, and tonic recommended for pyorrhea

ROSEMARY—used as an herbal hairwash and astringent; a fine hair conditioner. May prevent premature baldness.

ASPARAGUS—diuretic laxative, sedative

ONION—variously prescribed for earache and coughs

STRAWBERRIES—dentifrice and tooth whitener

BASIL—may calm nerves

...and that's just a peek into the pantry. Here is the book that will be your guide to a new adventure in healthful living that is fascinating, fun and good for what ails you!

D1067146

PROVEN HERBAL REMEDIES

JOHN H. TOBE

Edited and Abridged for the Modern Reader

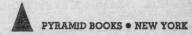 PYRAMID BOOKS • NEW YORK

PROVEN HERBAL REMEDIES

A PYRAMID BOOK

First printing, May 1973

ISBN 0-515-03029-5

Printed in the United States of America

Pyramid Books are published by Pyramid Communications, Inc. Its trademarks, consisting of the word "Pyramid" and the portrayal of a pyramid, are registered in the United States Patent Office.

PYRAMID COMMUNICATIONS, INC.
919 Third Avenue
New York, New York 10022, U.S.A.

DEDICATION

To all those men and women, wherever they are found on this earth, who believe in medical and healing freedom for all and who are willing to fight to the bitter end for this freedom, this volume is seriously dedicated.

It is my belief that no one should be forced to take or be injected with drugs of any kind; no one should be forced to undergo a blood transfusion, any more than anyone should be forced to undergo a heart or a kidney transplant operation.

I voice my profound admiration and respect for all those who have fought in the past and those who continue to fight so bravely in spite of continued persecution by over-zealous authorities.

CONTENTS

APOLOGIA

It has been the general practice now for some years, when offering other means of healing than organized medicine, to give or state a disclaimer... and the phrasing runs similar to this:

"The material, recipes, botanical materia medica compounds, infusions and decoctions in this book are not intended to replace the services of a physician or physicians. A physician should be consulted when the condition logically requires his services."

It has never been brought to my attention that such a statement or disclaimer is required or necessary by law. I would presume that this disclaimer was given to prevent legal action being taken against the author.

I hold no animosity towards the medical profession. In fact, I respect many members of this profession. But I do not in the slightest degree feel that they are the only, nor the best, nor the noblest profession in the healing arts.

I am not even slightly convinced that modern medicine, with the use of the thousands of synthetic drugs, has done one iota better in the treatment of disease than the herbalist and his herbs. In fact, it is absolutely true that while many or most drugs are harmful and create side effects—which are often more serious than the disease being treated—the herbalists do much better. I, for one, have never heard of a single instance of serious side effects from the use of prescribed herbs.

It is an acknowledged fact that a large percentage of all those hospitalized are there because of purely iatrogenic diseases.

Because I have seen so many members of various healing professions make the statement about consulting your doctor, I am led to believe that it is necessary for them to do so if they are to remain in practice. If this is compulsory according to the laws of the land, I of course, will have no alternative but to comply, and this article is, in fact, my compliance.

However, to the best of my knowledge, we still have freedom of the press and I boldly state that every human being holds an inherent right to select the method of healing or the healer of his choice.

I do not suggest that herbs are the only or even the best form of healing, but I do emphatically claim that herbalism is mankind's oldest form of healing.

I further maintain that each individual has the right to read, to study, to investigate and then decide on the method or kind of healing that he thinks is best suited to his needs.

Forthrightly I state, if your condition requires the attention of a surgeon, then of course that is where you should go for assistance. If you feel that the removal of a gland, a protuberance, an organ or any other part of your anatomy is necessary for your well-being, then of course the logical choice is a surgeon. If you feel that you desire to be inoculated, vaccinated, injected or treated by a medical practitioner, then by all means that is where you should go.

By the same token, if you believe that a chiropractor, an osteopath, a podiatrist, a naturopath, a spiritual healer, a fasting specialist, a psychiatrist or a herbalist will best fulfill your needs, then of course it should be your right or privilege to consult him.

It is not my intent at this time to enter into a discussion concerning the merits, the qualifications or the implications involved in comparing the various schools of healing. I simply categorically contend that each individual has the right to choose his mode or method of healing.

JOHN H. TOBE

Chiropractor
    - treatment of diease by
        manipulating the spine

Osteopath
    - treatment of diease by
        manipulating the bones &
        muscles.

Pediatrist
    -

Naturopath

Spiritual healer

Fasting

Psychiatrist

11

Herbalist

FORMS OF BOTANICAL
MEDICINAL PREPARATIONS

INFUSIONS

These preparations are generally made of ground or bruised roots, barks, herbs, or seeds, by pouring boiling water over the drug, letting it stand for half an hour, occasionally stirring, and finally straining the clear liquid carefully off. Sometimes cold water may be used, as in the case of a few bitters, such as Calumba, Quassia, etc., when the ground drug will be found to yield its properties to water without heat. The usual quantity of drug to 1 pint of water is 1 oz., but in a few cases where the drugs contain very active principles, less is sufficient. The dose of most infusions varies from a tablespoonful to a wineglassful or a teacupful.

DECOCTIONS

As a rule decoctions are made by pouring cold water upon the cut, bruised, or ground drug, the mixture being boiled for twenty minutes to half an hour, cooled and strained. Roots and barks are generally treated in this manner, as they need longer subjection to heat to extract their virtues. Decoctions are generally made in a strength of 1 oz. to 1 pt., but, as the water boils away, it is best to use 1½ pt., and the decoctions should then, when finished, measure 1 pt. The length of time depends upon the readiness with which the drug gives up its active principles to the liquid. The dose varies from two teaspoonfuls to a wineglassful or two.

LIQUID EXTRACTS

These are most popular and convenient preparations inasmuch as, if properly made, they are the most concentrated fluid forms in which vegetable drugs may be obtained. Liquid extracts are made in a variety of ways —evaporation by heat, in vacuo; cold percolation; high pressure, etc.—each drug being treated in that manner by which its properties may best be extracted and held in concentrated solution. The strength of a liquid extract is 1 in 1, or 1 oz. fluid represents 1 oz. of crude drug—for instance, 1 oz. of Liquid Ext. Golden Seal would represent the medicinal value of 1 oz. of Golden Seal Root. Liquid extracts are daily becoming more popular, and, as they may be easily obtained, bid fair to rival the tinctures and preparations which have made homeopathy so popular with those who seek an easy way of keeping a household stock of domestic remedies.

SOLID EXTRACTS

Are prepared by evaporating to the consistence of honey the fresh juices or strong infusions of vegetable drugs. They may also be manufactured by spirituous process, in which case the alcohol is recovered by means of distillation from a strong tincture of the drug. Solid extracts are employed chiefly in the manufacture of pills, plasters, ointments, and compressed tablets.

TINCTURES

Are spirituous preparations made with pure or diluted spirits of wine of drugs containing gummy, resinous, or volatile principles, or of any drugs rendered useless by the application of heat in any form, or of the great number of drugs which will not yield their properties to water alone, as their active principles are more readily extracted by spirit, better held in solution and preserved from deterioration.

Tinctures are generally made in a strength of 1 to 2 oz. of drug to 1 pt. The dose varies according to the active principles contained in the drug.

PILLS

Are perhaps the best known and most largely used form of medicines, chiefly because of their handy form and general convenience, and also because of their comparative tastelessness. Pills are for the most part composed of concentrated extracts and alkaloids in combination with active crude drugs. They may be obtained coated or uncoated, but the pearl-coated pill is the general favorite, as it is quite tasteless, and the coating, if properly made, is readily soluble in the stomach.

TABLETS

Are made by compressing drugs into a very small compass. It is claimed for them that they are superior to pills, because they are more easily administered and by reason of their rapid dissolution in the stomach are quicker in their action.

CAPSULES

Are gelatine containers of convenient sizes for swallowing and holding oils, balsams, etc., which, because of their nauseous taste or smell, would be difficult to administer. Such drugs as Cod Liver Oil, Castor Oil, Copaiba, Sandalwood Oil, etc., are largely given in this form, because objection is made to the remedies in their natural state.

SUPPOSITORIES

Are small cones made of some convenient and easily soluble base, and used where it is desired to apply medicines per rectum. They are invaluable in the treatment of internal piles, cancers, fistula, etc. They are also made of nutrient ingredients, and passed into the bowels where patients are unable to take nourishment in the usual manner.

PESSARIES

Are similar to suppositories, but are made in a suitable shape to be used in female complaints, where it is desirable to apply remedies to the walls of the internal passages.

CONCENTRATIONS

Are a class of medicinal resins or resinoids obtained from medicinal drugs by precipitation from their alcoholic preparations, either by water, distillation, or other suitable means.

Those at present in use contain one or more, but not always all the therapeutic virtues of the drugs from which they are made, and in many cases are only powdered extracts.

DEFINITIONS OF HERBAL MEDICAL TERMS

ALTERNATIVE: A medicine that alters the processes of nutrition and excretion, restoring the normal functions of the system.

ANODYNE: An agent that will relieve pain; milder in form than an analgesic.

ANTIBILIOUS: Relieving bilious conditions.

ANTIPHLOGISTIC: Capable of relieving inflammation.

ANTIPERIODIC: Antimalarial; preventing regular recurrences.

ANTISCORBUTIC: An agent effective against or a remedy for scurvy.

ANTISCROFULOUS: An agent effective against or a remedy for scrofula.

ANTISEPTIC: (a) Preventing decay, putrefaction, or sepsis. (b) An agent that will prevent the growth or arrest the development of microorganisms.

ANTISPASMODIC: (a) Relieving or checking spasm. (b) An agent that will relieve spasm.

APERIENT: A very mild laxative.

APHRODISIAC: An agent which stimulates sexual desire.

AROMATIC: (a) Having an agreeable odor. (b) Belonging to that series of carbon compounds in which the carbon atoms form closed rings (as in benzene) as distinguished from the aliphatic series in which the atoms form straight or branched chains.

ASTRINGENT: (a) Drawing together, constricting, binding. (b) An agent that has a constricting or binding effect, e.g., one which checks hemorrhages, secretion, etc.

BALSAMIC: (a) Pertaining to balsam. (b) Aromatic.

BITTER: Having a disagreeable taste.

CARDIAC: (a) Pertaining to the heart or to the cardiac orifice into the stomach. (b) Having heart disease. (c) A heart tonic.

CARMINATIVE: An agent that will remove gases from the gastrointestinal tract.

CATHARTIC: An active purgative, usually producing several evacuations which may or may not be accompanied by pain.

CORRECTIVE: (a) A drug that modifies action of another. (b) Pertaining to such a drug.

DEMULCENT: An agent that will soothe the part or soften the skin to which applied. The term is usually restricted to agents acting on mucous membrane.

DERMATIC: An agent effective against dermatitis or other skin conditions.

DETERGENT: (a) A medicine that purges or cleanses; cleansing. (b) A cleaning agent prepared synthetically from higher alcohols, sulfuric acid and caustic soda.

DIAPHORETIC: A sudorific or an agent which increases perspiration. The term sudorific is usually confined to those active agents that cause drops of perspiration to collect on the skin.

DIGESTIVE: An agent effective against digestive disorders; an aid to digestion.

DIURETIC: Increasing or an agent which increases the secretion of urine.

18

EMETIC: Medicine that induces vomiting.

EMOLLIENT: An agent that will soften and soothe the part when applied locally. The term is usually confined to agents affecting the surface of the body.

EXPECTORANT: An agent that facilitates the removal of the secretions of the bronchopulmonary mucous membrane. Expectorants are sometimes classed as sedative expectorants and stimulating expectorants.

HEMOSTATIC: (a) Checking hemorrhage. (b) Any substance which checks bleeding without being directly applied to the bleeding areas.

HEPATIC: Pertaining to the liver.

HYDROGOGUE: An agent for conveying water.

HYPNOTIC: (a) Pertaining to sleep or hypnosis. (b) An agent that induces sleep or which dulls the senses.

INSECTICIDE: (a) An agent used to exterminate insects. (b) Destructive to insects.

IRRITANT: An agent which, when used locally, produces more or less local inflammatory reaction. Anything which induces or gives rise to irritation.

LAXATIVE: A mildly purgative medicine; an aperient or mild cathartic producing one or two evacuations without pain.

MYOTIC: (a) An agent that will contract the pupil of the eye. (b) Producing contraction of a pupil.

NARCOTIC: (a) Producing stupor or sleep. (b) A drug which in moderate doses depresses the central nervous system thus relieving pain and producing sleep but which in excessive dose produces unconsciousness, stupor, coma, and possibly death. (c) Anything that soothes, relieves or lulls. (d) One addicted to the use of narcotics.

NERVINE: (a) Acting as a nerve sedative. (b) An agent that lessens irritability of nerves and increases nerve energy.

NUTRITIVE: Pertaining to the process of assimilating food; having the property of nourishing.

OXYTOCIC: (a) An agent which stimulates uterine contractions. (b) Accelerating childbirth.

PARASITICIDE: (a) Killing parasites. (b) An agent that will kill parasites.

PURGATIVE: (a) Cleansing. (b) An agent that will cause watery evacuation of the intestinal contents.

RESOLVENT: (a) Promoting disappearance of inflammation. (b) That which causes dispersion of inflammation.

STERNUTATORY: Causing sneezing.

STIMULANT: Any agent temporarily increasing functional activity.

STOMACHIC: (a) Concerning the stomach. (b) Medicine exciting action of the stomach.

STYPTIC: (a) Contracting a blood vessel; stopping a hemorrhage by astringent action. (b) Anything that checks a hemorrhage.

SUDORIFIC: (a) Secreting or promoting the secretion of sweat. (b) Agent which produces sweating.

TONIC: (a) Pertaining to or characterized by tension or contraction, especially muscular tension. (b) Restoring tone. (c) A medicine that increases strength and tone.

VERMIFUGE: Agent for expelling intestinal worms.

COMMON DOSES AND EQUIVALENTS

1 teaspoonful	1 dram
1 dessertspoonful	2 drams
1 tablespoonful	½ fluid ounce
1 wineglassful	1½-2 fluid ounces or 3-4 table-spoonfuls
1 teacupful	4-5 fluid ounces or 8-10 table-spoonfuls

ABBREVIATIONS FOR WEIGHTS AND MEASURES

cc.	cubic centimeter(s)
dr.	dram(s)
fl. dr.	fluid dram(s)
fl. oz.	fluid ounce(s)
ft.	foot (feet)
g.	gram(s)
gr.	grain(s)
in.	inch(es)
min.	minim(s)
oz.	ounce(s)
pt.	pint

TABLE OF WEIGHTS
AND MEASURES

1 grain	0.0648 grams
1 scruple (20 grains)	1.2959 "
1 dram (60 grains)	3.8879 "
1 ounce avoirdupois (437.5 grains)	28.3495 "
1 ounce Apothecaries' or Troy (480 grains)	31.1035 "
1 pound (7,000 grains)	453.59 "
	or 0.4356 kilograms
1 minim	0.0592 milliliters
1 fluid dram (60 minims)	3.5515 "
1 fluid ounce (8 drams)	28.4123 "
1 pint (20 ounces)	0.5682 liters
1 gallon (8 pints)	4.5459 "
1 meter	39.3701 inches
1 decimeter, 0.1 of meter	3.9370 "
1 centimeter, 0.01 of meter	0.3970 "
1 millimeter, 0.001 of meter	0.0397 "

ALPHABETICAL
LIST OF AILMENTS

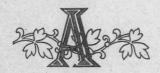

ACNE AND OTHER SKIN AFFLICTIONS

PLANT: Fumitory · *Fumaria officinalis*
WHERE FOUND: Europe and Asia
PART USED: Herb
ACTION: Aperient, diuretic, slightly tonic
USE: Mainly for stomach disorders and skin afflictions.
METHOD: Infusion of 1 oz. to 1 pt. of boiling water
DOSAGE: Wineglassful every 3 hours

ACUTE MANIA—MUSCULAR TWITCHING

PLANT: Hemlock · *Conium maculatum*
WHERE FOUND: Europe and Great Britain
PART USED: Leaves and unripe fruits
ACTION: Anodyne, sedative
USE: Recognized of particular service in all spasmodic conditions; e.g., chorea, acute mania and epilepsy. Good for whooping cough.
METHOD: From leaves, powdered leaves. From seeds, liquid extract.
DOSAGE: Powdered leaves, 2-8 gr.; Liquid extract, 2-5 min.

NOTE: An overdose can produce paralysis. Extremely dangerous and must be administered only by a qualified practitioner.

ACUTE TONSILITIS

PLANT: Hellebore, American   *Veratrum viride*
WHERE FOUND: Canada and the United States
PART USED: Rhizome
ACTION: Cardiac depressant
USE: An excellent remedy for acute tonsilitis, and as a gargle for sore throat. Most useful in febrile and inflammatory condition of the respiratory organs. Relieves irritation of the nervous system and is highly regarded as a remedy in convulsions, mania, neuralgia and headache. It is a known poison and should be used with care and caution.
METHOD: Powdered root
DOSAGE: 1 to 2 gr.

AGUE

PLANT: Calamus   *Acorus calamus*
WHERE FOUND: Throughout Europe and Britain
PART USED: Rhizome
ACTION: Aromatic, carminative, stomachic
USE: Recommended for flatulence, wind, colic, ague. An old remedy for ague. This root was known to the ancient Greek and Arabian doctors. The fresh candied root was used by the Indians and the Turks for dypepsia.
METHOD: Infusion of 1 oz. to 1 pt. boiling water
DOSAGE: Taken freely in teacupful doses

ALCOHOLISM

PLANT: Gold Thread   *Coptis trifolia*
WHERE FOUND: India. However the variety *groelandica,* which is equal in medicinal value, grows in Canada and the United States.
PART USED: Rhizome

26

ACTION: A decoction of Gold Thread will frequently destroy the desire for alcoholic beverages. A bitter tonic.
USE: Its excellent qualities should be better known. It improves the appetite, promotes digestion and acts as a general stimulant to the system. Highly beneficial in convalescence. Has been proven useful in chronic inflammation of the stomach. Soothes irritation of the mouth.
METHOD: Steep a teaspoonful of the powdered root in a cup of boiling water.
DOSAGE: Teaspoonful 4 or 5 times daily

ANEMIA

PLANT: Cicely, Sweet *Myrrhis odorata*
WHERE FOUND: Common British and European plant
PART USED: Herb, root
ACTION: Carminative, expectorant, stomachic
USE: The fresh root eaten freely has proven useful for coughs and flatulence, as well as a gentle stimulant in indigestion and stomach disorders. The dried root is best made into a decoction and the herb is best made into an infusion. An infusion made from the herb gives good results for anemia, and is a splendid tonic for young girls.
METHOD: Decoction of 1 oz. root to 1 pt. boiling water; infusion of 1 oz. herb to 1 pt. boiling water.

ANTISPASMODIC

PLANT: Cedron *Simaba cedron*
WHERE FOUND: Central America
PART USED: Seeds
ACTION: Antispasmodic, bitter, fever reducer, sedative, tonic
USE: The exceedingly bitter seeds have been used in malarial complaints, dyspepsia and intermittent fevers.
METHOD: Infusion of 1 oz. to 1 pt. boiling water
DOSAGE: 1 tablespoonful 3 or 4 times a day

APHRODISIAC

PLANT: Damiana   *Turnera diffusa*
WHERE FOUND: Sub-tropical America, Africa and Texas
PART USED: Leaves
ACTION: Aphrodisiac, diuretic, tonic
USE: Damiana is very largely prescribed on account of its aphrodisiac qualities, and there is no doubt that it has a very great general and beneficial action on the reproductive organs. It also acts as a tonic to the nervous system.
METHOD: Extract of Damiana
DOSAGE: 5 to 10 gr.

ARTHRITIS AND MALNUTRITION

PLANT: Lucerne or Alfalfa   *Medicago sativa*
WHERE FOUND: Europe and America; wherever cattle are raised.
PART USED: Whole herb.
ACTION: Alterative, nutritive
USE: Known generally as alfalfa. It is known best as one of the finest of all grasses for cattle. Its nutritive value has been recognized for centuries. Widely used for arthritis, where the powdered herb is taken with cider vinegar and honey: one teaspoonful of each in a glass of water. Has long been used as a strengthening and weight-adding tonic.

ARTICULAR STIFFNESS

PLANT: Poison Oak   *Rhus toxicodendron*
WHERE FOUND: North America
PART USED: Leaves
ACTION: Irritant, narcotic, stimulant
USE: Valuable in articular stiffness and acute rheumatism. Also has been used with success in the treatment of

obstinate skin diseases and in small doses is an excellent sedative for the nervous system.

METHOD: Liquid extract
DOSAGE: 5 to 30 drops

ASTHMA

PLANT: Butterbur *Petasites vulgaris*
WHERE FOUND: Europe and North Asia
PART USED: Root
ACTION: Cardiac, diuretic, stimulant, tonic
USE: Has long been in use as a remedy in fevers, asthma, colds and urinary complaints, gravel and plague. A stimulant for weak heart and good in dropsy.
METHOD: Decoction of 1 oz. in 1 pt. boiling water.
DOSAGE: Frequent wineglassful doses.

ATROPHY OF TESTES AND MAMMAE

PLANT: Saw Palmetto *Serenoa serrulata*
WHERE FOUND: Eastern North America
PART USED: Berry
ACTION: Diuretic, nutritive, sedative, tonic
USE: Has a marked effect on all the glandular tissues for it builds up strength and flesh rapidly. Should be used in atrophy of testes and mammae.
METHOD: Powdered berries
DOSAGE: 15 gr.

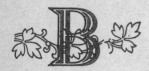

BARRENNESS AND PAIN RELIEVER

PLANT: Catnip   *Nepeta cataria*
WHERE FOUND: Native to England but found in North America
PART USED: Herb
ACTION: Carminative, diaphoretic, cooling, tonic
USE: Produces free perspiration, useful in colds, also relieves pains and flatulence.

Catnip gets its name from the liking of cats for this plant. It is said that when it starts to wither they will roll themselves in it and chew it. There is an old belief that it makes cats frolicsome, amorous and full of battle.
METHOD: Infusion of 1 oz. to 1 pt. boiling water
DOSAGE: For children: 2 or 3 teaspoonfuls; Adults: 2 tablespoonfuls.

BEAUTIFYING AGENT

PLANT: Frostwort or Rock Rose
                         Helianthemum canadense
WHERE FOUND: Europe, Great Britain and America
PART USED: Herb
ACTION: Alterative, astringent, tonic
USE: Taken internally as a remedy for scrofula. Used externally as a wash for ulcers and sores.
METHOD: Infusion of 1 oz. to 1 pt. boiling water
DOSAGE: Wineglassful doses taken freely

BILIARY CONCRETIONS

PLANT: Olive   *Olea europaea*
WHERE FOUND: Mediterranean lands
PART USED: Oil
ACTION: Aperient, emollient, nutritive.
USE: Through the ages it has been used internally as a remedy for bowel diseases, habitual constipation, lead colic, for removing worms, and in large doses dispels biliary concretions. Externally it forms an important role in embrocations, ointments and liniments, used in bruises, burns, scalds, rheumatic and skin ailments. Proven valuable as a soother for teething children, keeping the bowels regular and acting as a tonic by absorption.
METHOD: The best virgin oil should be obtained.
DOSAGE: From a teaspoonful to 2 tablespoonfuls as indicated

BLACK AND BLUE MARKS ON SKIN

PLANT: Bay Tree   *Laurus nobilis*
WHERE FOUND: Europe
PART USED: Leaves, fruits, oil
ACTION: Stomachic
USE: Opens obstructions of the liver, spleen, and other inward parts which cause jaundice, dropsy, etc. . . . The oil takes away the marks of the skin and flesh by bruises, falls, etc. and dissolves the congealed blood in them. It helps also the itch, scabs, and weals in the skin.

BLADDER, GRAVEL AND KIDNEY COMPLAINTS

PLANT: Parsley Piert   *Alchemilla arvensis*
WHERE FOUND: Europe
PART USED: Herb
ACTION: Demulcent, diuretic

USE: Long used in cases of gravel, kidney and bladder complaints. It acts directly on the parts affected, and will be found exceedingly valuable even in seemingly incurable cases.

METHOD: Infusion of 1 oz. herb to 1 pt. boiling water

DOSAGE: Teacupful doses three times a day

BLEEDING, TO STOP

PLANT: Love-Lies- Bleeding

Amaranthus hypochondriacus

WHERE FOUND: Native to Persia but widely cultivated everywhere

PART USED: Flowers and plant

ACTION: Astringent, corrective, hemostatic

USE: It is used externally as an application in ulcerated conditions; as a douche in leucorrhea; and as a wash for ulcers.

METHOD: Decoction

DOSAGE: Wineglassful doses as needed

BLEEDING OF MINOR WOUNDS

PLANT: Plantain   *Plantago major*

WHERE FOUND: Common weed almost everywhere

PART USED: Leaves

ACTION: Alterative, cooling, diuretic

USE: The fresh leaves will stop bleeding of minor wounds. When the fresh leaves are rubbed on parts of the body stung by insects or nettles, they will act as a coolant and give relief.

METHOD: Infusion of 1 oz. leaves to 1 pt. boiling water

DOSAGE: Wineglassful doses

BLISTERED SURFACES

PLANT: Mezereon   *Daphne mezereum*

WHERE FOUND: Native to the mountainous areas of Europe; cultivated in Great Britain

PART USED: Bark, root, root-bark
ACTION: Alterative, diuretic, stimulant
USE: Externally it is used as a lotion for blistered surfaces and indolent ulcers. Acts favorably in scrofula and rheumatism when taken internally.
METHOD: Decoction of ½ oz. powdered root-bark in 1 pt. of water
DOSAGE: Wineglassful doses

BLOOD IMPURITIES AND BURNS

PLANT: Burdock   *Arctium lappa*
WHERE FOUND: Europe
PART USED: Root, herb, fruit and seeds
ACTION: Alterative, diaphoretic, diuretic
USE: Considered the finest blood purifier in the botanical kingdom.
METHOD: Root and seed, either or both, taken as a decoction: 1 oz. to 1½ pts. of water, boiled down to 1 pt.
DOSAGE: Wineglassful 3 or 4 times a day

BLOOD IMPURITIES AND SCURVY

PLANT: Brooklime   *Veronica beccabunga*
WHERE FOUND: Throughout Europe, almost always near water and frequently in beds of watercress
PART USED: Herb
ACTION: Alterative, antiscorbutic, antiscrofulous, diuretic
USE: It is given in scurvy and impurities of the blood. Also claimed to have the ability to pulverize bladder stone and pass the gravel away.
METHOD: Infusion of 1 oz. of leaves to 1 pt. boiling water
DOSAGE: Frequent wineglassful doses

BODY HEAT GENERATOR—COLDNESS OF EXTREMITIES

PLANT: Bayberry   *Myrica cerifera*
WHERE FOUND: Widely distributed in America and Eurasia
PART USED: Bark
ACTION: Astringent, stimulant, tonic
USE: Said to be one of the most useful and beneficial herbs in botanic medicure.
METHOD: 1 oz. powdered bark to 1 pt. boiling water
DOSAGE: Drink when warm, as tea

BRONCHIAL, LARYNGEAL, PULMONARY INFECTIONS

PLANT: Sunflower   *Helianthus annuus*
WHERE FOUND: America, Europe, Asia
PART USED: Seeds, leaves
ACTION: Diuretic, expectorant
USE: For years this plant has been used in bronchial, laryngeal and pulmonary infections, coughs and colds.
METHOD: 2 oz. Sunflower seeds and 1 qt. water boiled down to 12 oz. and strained. Add 6 oz. gin and 6 oz. sugar.
DOSAGE: 1 to 2 teaspoonfuls frequently during the day

BRONCHITIS, BRONCHIAL PNEUMONIA AND PHTHISIS

PLANT: Cocillana   *Guarea rusbyi*
WHERE FOUND: South America, the eastern Andes
PART USED: Bark
ACTION: Expectorant
USE: Small doses act as an expectorant; large doses are emetic in action.
METHOD: Powdered bark
DOSAGE: 8 to 15 gr.

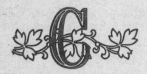

CARDIAC CONDITIONS

PLANT: Foxglove   *Digitalis purpurea*
WHERE FOUND: Europe and Great Britain, but grown everywhere in gardens
PART USED: Leaves
ACTION: Cardiac tonic, diuretic, sedative
USE: Digitalis is a poisonous plant and should be used with care and under proper supervision. Used in cardiac complaints arising from kidney diseases; also in dropsy and urinary suppression. Known to have cumulative action.
METHOD: Infusion of 1 dr. in 1 pt. boiling water
DOSAGE: Teaspoonful doses only as directed

CATARACT

PLANT: Willow, White   *Salix alba*
WHERE FOUND: Europe, Central Asia, North Africa
PART USED: Bark, leaves
ACTION: Antiperiodic, astringent, tonic
USE: Is very good for redness and dim eyesight and films that begin to grow over them.

CATARACT, LENTICULAR AND CAPSULAR

PLANT: Cineraria Maritima   *Senecio maritimus*
WHERE FOUND: Native to West Indies, but introduced

into most countries. Plants are readily available and are called Dusty Miller.

PART USED: Juice of the plant
ACTION: Unknown
USE: A trial is suggested before resorting to surgery.
METHOD: Juice of plant is sterilized
DOSAGE: Applied to the eye with an eye dropper

CATARRH

PLANT: Benne   *Sesamum indicum*
WHERE FOUND: Native to India; cultivated in warm climates
PART USED: Leaves
ACTION: Demulcent, laxative
USE: The fresh leaves are used in catarrhal conditions, diarrhea, dysentery, infections of kidney and bladder. The Indians steep a few leaves in water and drink the mucilaginous juice freely. Externally they use it for eye inflammation and skin complaints.
METHOD: Steep a few leaves in water
DOSAGE: Drink freely

CHAPPED HANDS

PLANT: Sanicle   *Sanicula europaea*
WHERE FOUND: Europe
PART USED: Herb
ACTION: Astringent, alterative
USE: To soften hands

CHEST, LUNG, STOMACH AND KIDNEY COMPLAINTS

PLANT: Balm of Gilead   *Populus candicans*
WHERE FOUND: Arabia
PART USED: Buds

ACTION: Diuretic, stimulant, sudorific, tonic
USE: This plant has been highly rated since time immemorial. The buds are used in making an ointment
used for all sorts of wounds, scalds, gout, piles and to
promote growth of hair. It has been used against gout,
rheumatism, bronchitis, intermittent fever and sciatics.
Balsamic odor and bitter taste.
METHOD: As an ointment massaged into the affected
parts

CHILDREN'S DIARRHEA

PLANT: Meadowsweet   *Spiraea ulmaria*
WHERE FOUND: Found in the meadows and woods of
Great Britain and Europe
PART USED: Herb
ACTION: Aromatic, astringent, diuretic
USE: Pleasant to the taste and widely used in herb beers.
Good remedy in strangury, dropsy and children's diar-
rhea, for which it is deemed a specific.
METHOD: Infusion of 1 oz. herb to 1 pt. boiling water
DOSAGE: Wineglassful doses as called for

CHRONIC INFECTIONS OF THE MUCOUS
AIR PASSAGES

PLANT: Galbanum   *Ferula galbaniflua*
WHERE FOUND: Persia and the Levant
PART USED: Gum-resin
ACTION: Stimulant, resolvent
USE: For ages it has been used internally in hysteria,
rheumatism and chronic infections of the mucous air
ointments.
METHOD: Emulsion
DOSAGE: 10-30 gr.

CHRONIC BRONCHITIS AND CATARRH

PLANT: Iceland Moss   *Cetraria islandica*
WHERE FOUND: Sweden, Central Europe
PART USED: Moss
ACTION: Demulcent, nutritive, tonic
USE: Normal dosage to improve both appetite and digestion. It does not cause constipation, but heavy usage may induce looseness of the bowels.
METHOD: Decoction of 1 oz. well washed moss to 1 pt. water
DOSAGE: 1 to 4 oz.

CHRONIC CONSTIPATION—INTESTINAL INDIGESTION

PLANT: Black Root   *Leptandra virginica*
WHERE FOUND: North America
PART USED: Rhizome
ACTION: Antiseptic, cathartic, diaphoretic, tonic
USE: Used mainly for its cathartic effect, for it acts with certainty and without griping. Invaluable in fevers, purifying the blood.
METHOD: Powder
DOSAGE: ¼ to 1 dr.

CHRONIC DISCHARGES OF BLOOD FROM THE UTERUS

PLANT: Saffron (Fall blooming)   *Crocus sativus*
WHERE FOUND: Asia Minor
PART USED: Flower pistils
ACTION: Carminative, diaphoretic
USE: It arrests chronic discharges of blood from the uterus. Also used in amenorrhea, dysmenorrhea and hysteria.
METHOD: Infusion of 1 dr. in 1 pt. boiling water
DOSAGE: Given in wineglassful to teacupful doses

CHRONIC IRRITATION OF THE MUCOUS MEMBRANE

PLANT: Mountain Laurel   *Kalmia latifolia*
WHERE FOUND: United States
PART USED: Leaves
ACTION: Alterative, astringent, cardiac sedative
USE: It is regarded as a most efficient remedy in overcoming obstinate chronic irritation of the mucous membrane.
METHOD: Decoction of 1 oz. of herb in 1 qt. water, boiled down to 1 pt.
DOSAGE: Tablespoonful doses

CHRONIC RHEUMATISM

PLANT: Guaiacum   *Guaiacum officinale*
WHERE FOUND: West Indies and South America
PART USED: Wood and resin
ACTION: Alterative, diaphoretic
USE: It is considered a valuable remedy for chronic rheumatism, gout and impurities in the blood. It is generally used in conjunction with sarsaparilla and is used in most blood-purifying compounds.
METHOD: Infusion of 1 oz. to 1 pt. boiling water
DOSAGE: Tablespoonful 3 or 4 times a day

COMMON COLD AND COLD SORES

PLANT: Dulse, True and Common
        Halymenia edulis and palmata
WHERE FOUND: Coast of Britain and New Brunswick
PART USED: Whole plant
ACTION: Corrective, purifying, nutritive, tonic, stimulant
USE: Does not induce thirst. One of the best balanced vegetable foods available. It is claimed that it contains more than 300 times more iodine than wheat and 50 times more iron. For the treatment of colds and cold

sores, its success is remarkable. Also a preventive of goiter.

METHOD: Eat the dried dulse as you would a stick of celery or a few leaves of lettuce.

DOSAGE: About half an ounce daily.

CONGESTIVE CHILLS AND INDIGESTION

PLANT: Pepper or Black Pepper   *Piper nigrum*

WHERE FOUND: Malabar and Travancore (India); also introduced to all other tropical areas

PART USED: Unripe berries

ACTION: Carminative, stimulant

USE: Pepper is considered a valuable gastrointestinal stimulant, of great service in flatulence, congestive chills and indigestion.

METHOD: Powdered peppercorns

DOSAGE: 3-15 gr.

CONSTIPATION

PLANT: Cassia Pods   *Cassia fistula*

WHERE FOUND: East and West Indies, Egypt

PART USED: Pulp

ACTION: Pleasant fruit laxative

USE: The pulp of Cassia is a gentle, soluble medicine, pleasant to take and purges very gently. It is usually combined with Senna or some other laxative.

DOSAGE: 60 to 120 gr.

CONSTIPATION

PLANT: Manna   *Fraxinus ornus*

WHERE FOUND: Southern Europe

PART USED: Concrete exudation

ACTION: Laxative, nutritive

USE: Considered useful as a laxative for infants, children and pregnant women.

METHOD: Combined with a laxative or carminative

DOSAGE: Teaspoonful up to 2 oz.

CONSTIPATION DUE TO THE INACTIVITY
OF THE LIVER

PLANT: Wahoo   *Euonymus atropurpureus*
WHERE FOUND: North America
PART USED: Bark and bark of root
ACTION: Alterative, laxative, tonic
USE: Valuable in liver disorders, especially those follow-
ing or accompanied by fever. It may be given with every
confidence for constipation due to inactivity of liver.
METHOD: Extract
DOSAGE: 1 to 2 gr.

CONVALESCENT FOOD

PLANT: Pot Barley   *Hordeum distichon*
WHERE FOUND: Worldwide, but native to Asia
PART USED: Seeds
ACTION: Demulcent, nutritive
USE: For children suffering from diarrhea, catarrhal in-
flammation of bowels. One of the world's oldest and most
widely used foods, especially in the Northern hemi-
sphere.
METHOD: Decoction of 2 oz. of washed barleycorns in
one pint of water.
DOSAGE: Take as desired

COUGH REMEDY

PLANT: Coltsfoot   *Tussilago farfara*
WHERE FOUND: Europe and Britain; grows in wet places
and near brooks and rivers
PART USED: Leaves and flowers
ACTION: Demulcent, expectorant
USE: Esteemed as the most popular of cough remedies.

41

Generally used with other herbs such as Horehound, Marshmallow, Ground Ivy and others.

METHOD: Decoction of 1 oz. leaves to 1 qt. water, boiled down to 1 pt.

DOSAGE: Teacupfuls sweetened with honey. The dried leaves, cut and rolled, are smoked like cigarettes in pulmonary conditions.

COUGHS, PAROXYSMAL, CONVULSIVE AND WHOOPING

PLANT: Chestnut   *Castanea sativa*
WHERE FOUND: Europe, Great Britain and America
PART USED: Leaves
ACTION: Astringent, tonic
USE: In many lands chestnut leaves are quite popular in treatment of ague and fever. However it is best known for its remedial benefits in paroxysmal or convulsive and whooping coughs, as well as other excitable and irritable ailments of the respiratory organs.

METHOD: Infusion of 1 oz. leaves in 1 pt. boiling water
DOSAGE: Tablespoonful to wineglassful doses, taken 3 to 4 times daily

CURE-ALL

PLANT: Horsetail   *Equisetum arcense*
WHERE FOUND: Grows most everywhere
PART USED: Herb
ACTION: Astringent, diuretic
USE: Recommended for dropsy, gravel and kidney complaints. The ashes of the plant are said to be used for acidity of the stomach and dyspepsia.

METHOD: Liquid extract
DOSAGE: ¼ to 1 dr.

CUTANEOUS TUMORS

PLANT: Sorrel   *Rumex acetosa*
WHERE FOUND: Europe
PART USED: Leaves
ACTION: Diuretic, cooling
USE: The following preparation is recommended for cutaneous tumors.
METHOD: Burnt Alum 1 dr.; Citric Acid 2 dr.; inspissated juice of Sorrel 1 oz.; water to 10 oz.
DOSAGE: Applied as a paint

CYSTITIS

PLANT: Marshmallow   *Althaea officinalis*
WHERE FOUND: Europe and Great Britain
PART USED: Leaves and root
ACTION: Demulcent, emollient
USE: In painful complaints of urinary organs and cystitis it exerts a relaxing effect upon the passages as well as acting as a curative. The powdered or crushed fresh roots make a good poultice, which may be relied upon to remove the most obstinate inflammation, and bring relief. The addition of Slippery Elm is an advantage and it should be applied to the part as hot as can be borne, renewing poultice when dry.
METHOD: An infusion of 1 oz. leaves to 1 pt. boiling water
DOSAGE: Wineglassful doses taken frequently

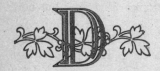

DIABETES AND ASTHMA

PLANT: Jaborandi   *Pilocarpus microphyllus*
WHERE FOUND: Brazil
PART USED: Leaves
ACTION: Diaphoretic, expectorant, stimulant
USE: Considered specially useful in diabetes and asthma.
METHOD: Infusion of 1 oz. leaves to 1 pt. boiling water
DOSAGE: Frequent mouthfuls

DIARRHEA AND DYSENTERY

PLANT: Blackberry, American   *Rubus villosus*
WHERE FOUND: North America; also in Europe
PART USED: Root and leaves
ACTION: Astringent, tonic
USE: A valuable remedy for diarrhea and dysentery.
METHOD: Infusion of 1 oz. root or leaves to 1 pt. water
DOSAGE: Taken in wineglassful doses.

DIMMING VISION AND EYE INFLAMMATION

PLANT: Cornflower   *Centaurea cyanus*
WHERE FOUND: Found growing wild in cornfields; also common garden plant
PART USED: Flowers
ACTION: Stimulant and tonic
USE: Said to be an excellent remedy for the inflammation of the eyes and dimness of eyesight.
METHOD: Infusion of 1 oz. to 1 pt. water
DOSAGE: Wineglassful as required

DIPHTHERIA AND CROUP

PLANT: Papaya   *Carica papaya*
WHERE FOUND: Native to tropical America, but now grown in all tropical lands
PART USED: Papain, prepared from the juice of the unripe fruit and leaves
ACTION: Digestive
USE: The digestive enzyme papain is administered widely in various digestive disorders where albuminoid substances pass away undigested. It is generally used in combination with an alkali, such as bicarbonate of soda, and acts best in an alkaline medium. A solution of the enzyme (ferment) is claimed to dissolve the false membranes in diptheria and croup, when applied frequently.
METHOD: Papain
DOSAGE: 2 to 10 gr.

DROPSY

PLANT: Toadflax, Yellow   *Linaria vulgaris*
WHERE FOUND: Europe
PART USED: Herb
ACTION: Astringent, detergent, hepatic
USE: A good application for piles is an ointment made from the fresh plant. As an alterative in jaundice, liver, skin diseases and scrofula.
METHOD: Infusion of 1 oz. herb to 1 pt. boiling water
DOSAGE: Take wineglassful doses as desired

DRUNKENNESS

PLANT: Wood Betony   *Stachys betonica*
WHERE FOUND: Europe
PART USED: Herb
ACTION: Alterative, aromatic, astringent

USE: It is said to hinder drunkenness if taken before-hand and quickly to expel it afterwards. The root is not used in medicine. It has an obnoxious flavor and induces vomiting.

DRY COUGHS

PLANT: Licorice or Liquorice　　　*Glycyrrhiza glabra*
WHERE FOUND: Mediterranean Europe
PART USED: Root
ACTION: Demulcent, emollient
METHOD: Here is a recipe used with much success by one Dr. Malone of London:

Take a large teaspoonful of Linseed, 1 oz. of Liquorice Root, and ¼ lb. of best raisins. Put them into 2 quarts of soft water and simmer down to 1 quart. Then add to it ¼ lb. brown sugar candy and tablespoonful of white wine vinegar or lemon juice. Drink ½ pint when going to bed and take a little whenever the cough is troublesome.

N.B. It is best to add the vinegar to that quantity which is required for immediate use.

DYSENTERY

PLANT: Bael　　　　　　　　　　*Aegle marmelos*
WHERE FOUND: India
PART USED: Fruit, unripe and dried
ACTION: Astringent, laxative
USE: This is an Indian remedy and is considered prac-tically a specific for diarrhea and dysentery in that country. It is claimed that it never constipates.
METHOD: Liquid extract. Also used in the form of a decoction or jelly.
DOSAGE: 60-120 min.

DYSMENORRHEA (Painful Menstruation)

PLANT: Pulsatilla   *Anemone pulsatilla*
WHERE FOUND: Europe and Asia
PART USED: Herb
ACTION: Alterative, antispasmodic, nervine
USE: Highly valued as a remedy for nervous exhaustion in women, especially when due to menstrual difficulties. Has a stimulating effect on all mucous surfaces. Valuable in catarrh, amenorrhea and other conditions.
METHOD: Fluid extract
DOSAGE: 2 to 5 drops every few hours during the day prior to the expected period

DYSPEPSIA

PLANT: Centaury   *Erythraea centaurium*
WHERE FOUND: Europe and British heaths
PART USED: Herb, leaves
ACTION: Aromatic, bitter, stomachic, tonic
USE: Most used in dyspepsia. Also used in conjunction with Barberry bark for jaundice.
METHOD: Infusion of 1 oz. to 1 pt. boiling water
DOSAGE: Wineglassful as desired

DYSPEPSIA

PLANT: Galangal   *Alpinia officinarum*
WHERE FOUND: Island of Hainan and also along the coast of southeast China
PART USED: Rhizome
ACTION: Carminative, stimulant
USE: The powdered rhizome is used as a snuff. The decoction is of great value in dyspepsia, for preventing fermentation and easing flatulence.
METHOD: Decoction of 1 oz. to 1 pt. boiling water
DOSAGE: Tablespoonful to wineglassful doses, as preferred. Powdered root is used in pinches as snuff.

47

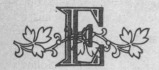

ECZEMA

PLANT: Celandine   *Chelidonium majus*
WHERE FOUND: Europe and English gardens
PART USED: Herb
ACTION: Alterative, diuretic, purgative
USE: Long used for eczema, scrofulous diseases, jaundice. The fresh juice is excellent when applied to corns and warts.
METHOD: Infusion of 1 oz. herb to 1 pt. boiling water
DOSAGE: Wineglassful doses as needed

ELEPHANTIASIS

PLANT: Calotropis   *Calotropis procera*
WHERE FOUND: India
PART USED: Bark
ACTION: Sudorific, tonic
USE: In India it is used as a local remedy for elephantiasis, leprosy and chronic eczema. Internally for diarrhea and dysentery.
METHOD: Powdered bark
DOSAGE: 3 to 10 gr. as an expectorant

ELIXIR

PLANT: Slippery Elm   *Ulmus fulva*
WHERE FOUND: North and Central America
PART USED: Inner bark

ACTION: Demulcent, diuretic, emollient

USE: The coarse powder forms the finest poultice to be obtained for all inflamed surfaces, ulcers, wounds, burns, boils, skin diseases, purulent ophthalmia, chilblains, etc. It soothes the part, disperses the inflammation, draws out impurities, and heals speedily.

METHOD: The food or gruel should be made as follows: Take a teaspoonful of the powder, mix well with the same quantity of powdered sugar and add 1 pt. of boiling water slowly, mixing as it is poured on. This may be flavored with cinnamon or nutmeg to suit the taste, and makes a very wholesome and sustaining food for infants.

DOSAGE: Inflammation in the bowels of infants and adults has been cured, when all other remedies have failed, by an injection into the bowels of an infusion of 1 oz. of powdered bark to 1 pt. of boiling water, used while warm.

ENERGESIS

PLANT: Yerba Mate or Paraguay Tea   *Ilex paraguensis*

WHERE FOUND: Paraguay, Brazil and other South American countries

PART USED: Leaves, and also the finely ground stems

ACTION: Diuretic, stimulant

USE: It is claimed that the natives can do a real hard day's work with nothing but frequent cups of strong Mate. General action similar to coffee or tea but much more stimulating, so its users claim. Does have antiscorbutic qualities. Recommended for rheumatism and gout.

METHOD: Infusion as tea—a teaspoonful to a cup of boiling water.

DOSAGE: Take as desired

ENFEEBLED STOMACH AND INTESTINES

PLANT: Canella   *Canella alba*
WHERE FOUND: West Indies
PART USED: Bark
ACTION: Antiscorbutic, aromatic, stimulant, tonic
USE: Useful in enfeebled conditions of the stomach and intestines. Used as a condiment by the natives of the West Indies.
METHOD: Pulverized bark
DOSAGE: 3 to 10 gr.

ENLARGEMENT OF SPLEEN

PLANT: Hedge-Hyssop   *Gratiola officinalis*
WHERE FOUND: Boggy places in the English countryside
PART USED: Herb, root
ACTION: Cathartic, diuretic, emetic
USE: Recommended in enlargement of the spleen, chronic infections of the liver and jaundice. It has also proven itself valuable in dropsical complaints. Large doses induce vomiting and purging.
METHOD: Infusion of ½ oz. powdered root to 1 pt. boiling water
DOSAGE: Tablespoonful doses as indicated

EPILEPSY

PLANT: Peony   *Paeonia officinalis*
WHERE FOUND: China and Tibet, but today a common and beautiful garden flower
PART USED: Root
ACTION: Antispasmodic, tonic
METHOD: Take the root of the male peony washed clean and stamped small and infuse it in sack for twenty-four hours at least; afterwards strain it, and take, morning and evening.

EYE DISEASES

PLANT: Quince   *Cydonia oblongata*
WHERE FOUND: Persia, but planted in Europe and America
PART USED: Seeds
ACTION: Demulcent, mucilaginous
USE: Externally it is used in eye diseases as a soothing lotion.

EYE DISORDERS

PLANT: Eyebright   *Euphrasia officinalis*
WHERE FOUND: Europe and Britain
PART USED: Herb
ACTION: Astringent and slightly tonic
USE: Its principal use is in treatment of the eyes: diseases of sight, weakness of vision and ophthalmia. An excellent lotion for general disorders of the eye is made in combination with Golden Seal.
METHOD: Liquid extract
DOSAGE: 1 dr.

EYE TROUBLES

PLANT: Clary   *Salvia sclarea*
WHERE FOUND: Found throughout Europe and the British Isles
PART USED: Herb, seed
ACTION: Antispasmodic and balsamic
USE: It is most useful and efficacious in any complaint of the eyes. Has also given relief in kidney diseases. Valued also as a stomachic in digestive troubles.
METHOD: Decoction of 1 oz. herb to 1 pt. boiling water
DOSAGE: Wineglassful twice daily

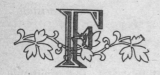

FEBRILE DISEASES

PLANT: Tamarinds *Tamarindus indica*
WHERE FOUND: Native to central Africa; cultivated in West Indies, India and East Indies
PART USED: Fruit, pulp
ACTION: Laxative, nutritive, cooling
USE: Considered an agreeable cooling drink in febrile diseases when used in small quantities and diluted with water.
METHOD: 1 oz. pulp boiled in 1 pt. milk and then strained.
DOSAGE: 2 to 4 drams

FEVERS

PLANT: Balm *Melissa officinalis*
WHERE FOUND: Widely planted in gardens, but native to Eurasia
PART USED: Herb
ACTION: Carminative, diaphoretic, cooling
USE: Induces mild perspiration, and also makes a pleasant and cooling tea for feverish patients. Considered a most useful herb either alone or in combination with others.
METHOD: 1 oz. herb in 1 pt. boiling water, allow to cool and then strain
DOSAGE: Drink freely

FEVERS (Intermittent)

PLANT: Berberis   *Berberis aristata*
WHERE FOUND: Native to India
PART USED: Stem
ACTION: Cooling, tonic
USE: Used in India as a bitter tonic in intermittent fevers.
METHOD: Powder
DOSAGE: 10 to 60 gr.

FEVERS (Including Malaria)

PLANT: Cinchona   *Cinchona officinalis*
WHERE FOUND: The Andes in South America
PART USED: Bark
ACTION: Antiperiodic, astringent, cooling, tonic
USE: A much esteemed herb in all typhoid and febrile conditions, and also for recurring and intermittent fevers. Highly rated as a general tonic and in debility, dyspepsia and neuralgia.
METHOD: Powdered bark
DOSAGE: 5 to 15 gr.

FRECKLES, SPOTS AND PIMPLES ON THE FACE

PLANT: Silverweed   *Potentilla anserina*
WHERE FOUND: Europe and Great Britain
PART USED: Herb
ACTION: Astringent, tonic
USE AND METHOD: Gerard writes: "The distilled water takes away freckles, spots, pimples in the face, and sunburning, but the herb, laid to infuse or steep in white wine is far better: but the best of all is to steep it in strong white wine vinegar, the face being often bathed or washed therewith."

GALL STONES

PLANT: Fringetree   *Chionanthus virginica*
WHERE FOUND: Southern United States
PART USED: Bark of root
ACTION: Alterative, diuretic, tonic
USE: It acts quickly and efficiaciously in liver complaints
as well as in jaundice and gall stones. In female disorders
it is beneficial in conjunction with Pulsatilla and other
remedies.
METHOD: Infusion of 1 oz. to 1 pt. boiling water. May
be used externally as a lotion or injection.
DOSAGE: Tablespoonful to wineglassful doses, as suited

GASTRIC IRRITATION AND CONGESTION

PLANT: Peach   *Prunus persica*
WHERE FOUND: Native to Persia and China, now widely
grown
PART USED: Bark, leaves and oil pressed from the seeds
ACTION: Diuretic, expectorant, sedative
USE: It has been found almost a specific for irritation
and congestion of gastric surfaces. Used also in coughs,
whooping cough and chronic bronchitis.
METHOD: Infusion of ½ oz. of bark or 1 oz. of leaves
to 1 pt. of boiling water
DOSAGE: Teaspoonful to a wineglassful as desired

GLANDULAR ENLARGEMENT

PLANT: Ivy   *Hedera helix*
WHERE FOUND: Native to Europe and Britain, but grown in most gardens
PART USED: Leaves, berries
ACTION: Cathartic, diaphoretic, stimulant
USE: Externally the leaves have been employed as poultices or fomentations in glandular enlargements, indolent ulcers and abscesses. It is claimed that a vinegar of these berries was used extensively during the London plague.

GOITER

PLANT: Kelp, Pacific   *Macrocystis pyrifera*
WHERE FOUND: Coast of California
PART USED: Whole plant
ACTION: Alterative, corrective, nutritive, tonic
USE: Said to prevent common goiter. Also of value in its treatment; considered an excellent source of iodine. Dried kelp contains about ten times as much iodine as the same amount of iodized salt. An excellent substitute for salt. Contains a wide variety of elements and nutrients highly regarded by health-minded people.
METHOD: Used as a condiment as you would table salt
DOSAGE: Daily with meals

GRANULAR CONJUNCTIVITIS

PLANT: Poke Root   *Phytolacca decandra*
WHERE FOUND: North America
PART USED: Root, berries
ACTION: Alterative, cathartic, emetic
USE: It has for many years been used in the treatment of granular conjunctivitis. Also considered a valuable

remedy in scabies, ulcers, ringworm, chronic rheumatism, dysmenorrhea and dyspepsia. The berries are considered milder in action than the root.

METHOD AND DOSAGE: Liquid extract, berries—½ to 1 dr.; Powdered root—1 to 5 gr.

GRAVEL AND DROPSY

PLANT: Bilberry   *Vaccinium myrtillus*
WHERE FOUND: Europe; likes boggy locations
PART USED: Ripe fruits
ACTION: Astringent, diuretic, cooling
USE: Of proven benefit in dropsy and gravel.
METHOD: Decoction of 1 oz. in 1 pt. boiling water
DOSAGE: Taken in tablespoonful or wineglassful doses as required

GRAVES DISEASE (Erophthalmic Goiter)

PLANT: Speedwell   *Veronica officinalis*
WHERE FOUND: Europe
PART USED: Herb
ACTION: Alterative, diuretic, expectorant
USE: Especially recommended in Graves disease and nephritis, opens all obstructions, promotes the menses. Know as a remedy against coughs, asthma and lung diseases.
METHOD: Infusion of 2 oz. in 1 pt. boiling water
DOSAGE: Small wineglassful doses as required

GUMS, INFECTIONS OF THE

PLANT: Columbine, Common   *Aquilegia vulgaris*
WHERE FOUND: Southern France
PART USED: Seeds
ACTION: Antiphlogistic
USE: The seeds operate by sweat and urine, open ob-

structions of the viscera, and are good for jaundice, for fevers, smallpox and measles as they throw out the pustules. A decoction of the leaves is good for sore throats, and a tincture of the flowers in brandy is recommended as an excellent gargle for scorbutic infection of the gums.

GUM STRENGTHENER

PLANT: Water Dock   *Rumex aquaticus*
WHERE FOUND: Europe
PART USED: Root
ACTION: Alterative, purifying, detergent
USE: Valuable remedy for cleansing ulcers of the mouth. As a powder it has detergent effects on the teeth. The root finely powdered has been recommended as an excellent dentifrice to strengthen the gums.
METHOD: Infusion of 1 oz. root to 1 pt. boiling water
DOSAGE: Wineglassful doses

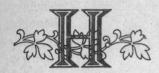

HAY FEVER AND ASTHMA

PLANT: Ephedra or Ma Huang   *Ephedra sinica*
WHERE FOUND: Northern China
PART USED: Stems
ACTION: Reduces susceptibility to hay fever and asthma
USE: It is claimed to have been used by the Chinese for thousands of years for asthmatic afflictions and bouts of hay fever. Ephedrine, the alkaloid, is the chief constituent.
METHOD: Liquid extract of Ephedrine
DOSAGE: ¼ to 1 dr.

HEAD WASH

PLANT: Fenugreek   *Trigonella foenum-graecum*
WHERE FOUND: North Africa and India
PART USED: Seeds
ACTION: Emollient
USE: Used externally as a poultice in abscesses, boils and carbuncles. Taken internally for inflamed conditions of stomach and intestines.
METHOD: Decoction of 1 oz. of seeds in 1 pt. water
DOSAGE: Teacupful doses as desired

HEARTBURN

PLANT: Spearmint   *Mentha viridis*
WHERE FOUND: Worldwide
PART USED: Herb, oil
ACTION: Antispasmodic, carminative, hepatic, stimulant
USE: Excellent for adding to other herbs to improve
both their action and flavor.
METHOD: Infusion of 1 oz. to 1 pt. boiling water.
Sweeten with honey for infants.
DOSAGE: Wineglassful doses or less, as needed

HEART DISORDERS

PLANT: Hawthorn   *Crataegus oxycantha*
WHERE FOUND: Grows wild in woodlands in America
and Great Britain
PART USED: Dried berries
ACTION: Cardiac, tonic
USE: These berries are claimed to be a curative remedy
for organic and functional heart disorders such as dysp-
noea, rapid and feeble heart action, hypertrophy, valvular
insufficiency and heart oppression.
METHOD: Liquid extract
DOSAGE: 10 to 15 drops taken 3 or 4 times a day

HEPATIC TORPOR AND CATARRH
OF THE BLADDER

PLANT: Boldo   *Peumus boldus*
WHERE FOUND: Chile
PART USED: Leaves
ACTION: Antiseptic, diuretic, liver stimulant
USE: Used chiefly against rheumatic pains, gall and
bladder conditions; also in chronic hepatic torpor and
dyspepsia.
METHOD: Liquid extract
DOSAGE: ⅛ to ½ dr.

59

HOARSENESS

PLANT: Hedge Mustard   *Sisymbrium officinale*
WHERE FOUND: Europe and Great Britain
PART USED: Herb
ACTION: Cooling, sedative
USE: A remedy for hoarseness and weak lungs. It is claimed to be an excellent aid in recovering the voice.
METHOD: Liquid extract
DOSAGE: ½ to 1 fl. dr.

HYSTERIA

PLANT: Skullcap   *Scutellaria laterifolia*
WHERE FOUND: North America
PART USED: Herb
ACTION: Antispasmodic, astringent, nervine, tonic
USE: Claimed by herbalists to be the finest nervine ever discovered. It is suggested that it be prescribed wherever disorders of the nervous system exist.
METHOD: Infusion of 1 oz. herb to 1 pt. boiling water
DOSAGE: Half a teacupful frequently.

HYSTERIA AND NERVOUS AFFLICTIONS
(Female)

PLANT: Chamomile   *Anthemis nobilis*
WHERE FOUND: Belgium, France and England; and of broad distribution
PART USED: Herb and flowers
ACTION: Antispasmodic, stomachic, tonic
USE: Very old renowned herb used for many centuries. Has been proven efficacious and is best known for its use in hysteria and nervous complaints of women. Makes a superior poultice when combined with crushed poppy

heads for relieving various pains and aches. Also used externally for neuralgia, toothache and earache.

METHOD: Infusion of 1 oz. to 1 pt. boiling water

DOSAGE: From a tablespoonful to a wineglassful

HYSTERICAL COMPLAINTS

PLANT: Camphor   *Cinnamomum camphora*

WHERE FOUND: Central China and Japan

PART USED: Distillation of Camphor wood chips

ACTION: Anodyne, vermifuge, antispasmodic, diaphoretic, sedative

USE: Internally it is used in cold chills. It has been found of great value in all inflammatory infections, fever and hysterical complaints. It also acts beneficially in gout, rheumatic pains and neuralgia. It is highly valued in all irritation of sexual organs. Externally, it can be safely applied in all cases of inflammation, bruises and sprains.

METHOD: Oil of Camphor

DOSAGE: 2 to 5 gr.

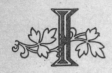

INFANTILE CONVULSIONS, TEETHING
AND OTHER AILMENTS

PLANT: Chamomile, German   *Metricaria chamomilla*
WHERE FOUND: Most parts of Europe, the British Isles
and elsewhere
PART USED: Flowers
ACTION: Carminative, sedative, tonic
USE: Excellent remedy in children's ailments. Of benefit
to the nerves (sedative) and tonic for the gastrointes-
tinal tract. Most useful during teething, for neuralgic
pains, stomach upsets, earache and infantile convulsions.
Externally used as a poultice.
METHOD: Inferior
DOSAGE: Give children freely in teaspoonful doses.

INFANTS' CORDIAL

PLANT: Peppermint   *Mentha piperita*
WHERE FOUND: All over Europe and North America
PART USED: Herb and oil (distilled)
ACTION: Carminative, stimulant, stomachic
USE: An old remedy for allaying nausea, flatulence,
sickness, vomiting and as an infants' cordial.
METHOD: Infusion of 1 oz. herb to 1 pt. boiling water
DOSAGE: Wineglassful doses

INFLAMMATORY DISEASES

PLANT: Abscess Root   *Polemonium reptans*
WHERE FOUND: Northern Europe
PART USED: Rhizome
ACTION: Alterative, astringent, diaphoretic, expectorant
USE: Used in febrile, inflammatory diseases, pleurisy, coughs, colds, bronchial and lung disorders.
METHOD: Infusion of 1 oz. to 1 pt. boiling water
DOSAGE: Wineglassful doses, preferably warm

INGROWING TOENAILS

PLANT: Amadou   *Polyporus fomentarius*
WHERE FOUND: Europe and Great Britain
PART USED: A hoof-shaped, obliquely triangular, sessile fungus. The inner part is composed of short tubular fibers arranged in layers.
ACTION: Hemostatic, styptic
USE: Amadou, known as Surgeon's Agaric, has been used for ages for arresting local hemorrhages. It is applied with pressure to the affected part.
METHOD: It is prepared for use by being cut into slices, chopped and beaten, soaked in a solution of niter, and allowed to dry. Then insert it between the nail and flesh.

INTERMITTENT AND RECURRING FEVERS

PLANT: Canadian Hemp   *Apocynum cannabinum*
WHERE FOUND: North America
PART USED: Root and rhizome
ACTION: Diaphoretic, diuretic, emetic, expectorant
USE: Recommended favorably in intermittent and recurring fevers. Useful in amenorrhea and leucorrhea.
METHOD: Decoction of 1 oz. to 1 pt. water
DOSAGE: Taken in tablespoonful doses frequently

INTESTINAL LUBRICANT

PLANT: Psyllium   *Plantago psyllium*
WHERE FOUND: South Europe
PART USED: Seeds
ACTION: Mucilaginous, bulking agent
USE: The seeds swell into a gelatinous mass when moistened, which stimulates and lubricates the intestinal tract.
METHOD: Place the psyllium in a glass and add warm water. Then stir until the mixture thickens, and then drink. Add a trace of fresh juice to make it palatable.
DOSAGE: Adult dose—2 to 4 teaspoonfuls after meals

INTESTINAL WORMS

PLANT: Butternut   *Juglans cinerea*
WHERE FOUND: North America
PART USED: Inner bark
ACTION: Cathartic, tonic, vermifuge
USE: A gentle purgative which does not bind after working. Also a remedy for worms in children.
METHOD: Make a syrup of ½ oz. of extract to 8 oz. simple syrup, beating well together in a mortar
DOSAGE: 1 tablespoonful of syrup twice daily

INWARD AND OUTWARD WOUNDS

PLANT: Self-Heal   *Prunella vulgaris*
WHERE FOUND: Europe
PART USED: Herb
ACTION: Astringent
USE: An old German saying is that "He needs neither physician nor surgeon that hath Self-Heal to help himself."

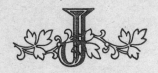

JAUNDICE, FEMALE OBSTRUCTIONS AND SCROFULOUS TUMORS

PLANT: Butcher's Broom   *Ruscus aculeatus*
WHERE FOUND: In the thickets in Britain
PART USED: Root, herb
ACTION: Aperient, purifying, diaphoretic, diuretic, laxative, sudorific
USE: Will be found useful in jaundice, gravel and female obstructions. Excellent results have been obtained by using the powdered root externally in cases of scrofulous tumors and ulcers.
METHOD: Decoction of 1 oz. to 1 pt. boiling water
DOSAGE: Wineglassful three or four times a day

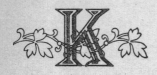

KIDNEY, SPLEEN, LIVER DISEASES, AND URINARY COMPLAINTS

PLANT: Dodder *Cuscuta epithymum*
WHERE FOUND: A parasitic plant found universally
PART USED: Herb
ACTION: Hepatic, laxative
METHOD: Infusion of 1 oz. of herb to 1 pt. boiling water
DOSAGE: Two to three teaspoonfuls twice daily

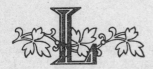

LARYNGITIS

PLANT: Pine Oils
Abies sibirica, Pinus mugo, Pinus sylvestris
WHERE FOUND: Europe and North America
PART USED: Oils
ACTION: Antiseptic, expectorant, inhalant
USE: Above oils are widely used as inhalations for bronchitis and laryngitis. Also used in obstinate coughs and other chest conditions. Used as an ointment for eczema and other skin ailments. May cause redness of skin.
METHOD: Apply oil to the affected parts

LETHARGY

PLANT: Thyme, Wild or Mother of Thyme
Thymus serpyllum
WHERE FOUND: Europe, West Asia and North Africa
PART USED: Herb
ACTION: Antispasmodic, carminative, tonic
USE: For convulsive coughs, whooping coughs, catarrh and sore throat.
METHOD: Infusion of 1 oz. herb to 1 pt. boiling water, sweetened with sugar or honey and made demulcent by Linseed or Acacia
DOSAGE: Tablespoonful doses frequently during the day

LIVER AND KIDNEY DISORDERS

PLANT: Dandelion   *Taraxacum officinale*
WHERE FOUND: Everywhere; considered a pest and weed
PART USED: Root and leaves
ACTION: Aperient, diuretic, tonic
USE: It is probably one of the most prescribed remedies on earth. It can be taken in any of many forms but it is claimed that its most beneficial action is best obtained in mixtures with other herbs. Chiefly used for liver and kidney disorders.
METHOD: The most pleasant way of taking this herb is in the form of a substitute for coffee. The roasted roots are ground and used as ordinary coffee, giving a beverage tasting much like the original article, and which certainly possesses most beneficial properties in cases of dyspepsia, gout, and rheumatism.

LIVER AND SPLEEN CONGESTION

PLANT: Bearsfoot, American   *Polymnia uvedalia*
WHERE FOUND: North America
PART USED: Root
ACTION: Anodyne, laxative, stimulant
USE: It has been successfully used in congestion of the liver and spleen, enlarged womb, inflamed glands and dyspepsia. Used externally as a hair tonic or in the form of an ointment.
METHOD: Liquid extract
DOSAGE: 15 to 60 drops

LIVER AND SPLEEN OBSTRUCTIONS

PLANT: Hartstongue   *Scolopendrium vulgare*
WHERE FOUND: Found in the woodlands of Britain; also a garden plant
PART USED: Herb
ACTION: Diuretic, laxative
USE: Specially recommended for removing obstructions from the liver and spleen; also proven for removing gravelly deposits in the bladder.
METHOD: Decoction of 2 oz. to 1 pt. of water
DOSAGE: A wineglassful, as needed

LIVER ENLARGEMENT

PLANT: Chicory   *Cichorium intybus*
WHERE FOUND: Popular garden plant in Great Britain and America; also grown commercially in Europe
PART USED: Root
ACTION: Diuretic, laxative, tonic
USE: A decoction freely taken has proven effective in liver enlargement, gout and rheumatic complaints. This is the same root used in coffee mixtures, when roasted and ground.
METHOD: Decoction of 1 oz. root to 1 pt. boiling water
DOSAGE: Taken freely

LOCKJAW

PLANT: White Pond Lily   *Nymphaea odorata*
WHERE FOUND: North America
PART USED: Root
ACTION: Antiseptic, astringent, demulcent
USE: Valuable as a gargle for mouth and throat, and wash for sore eyes, ophthalmia and lockjaw. Good in bowel disorders. The powdered root combined with

crushed linseed and powdered slippery elm makes a superb poultice. A decoction is used externally as an excellent lotion for bad legs and sores.

METHOD: Decoction of 1 oz. of root boiled for twenty minutes in 1 pt. of water

DOSAGE: Taken internally in wineglassful doses

LOOSE TEETH

PLANT: Pomegranate   *Punica granatum*
WHERE FOUND: Asia, the Caspian, the Persian Gulf, and the Mediterranean areas
PART USED: Fruit, rind of the fruit, bark of root, bark of stem
USE: Pomegranate is useful to strengthen the gums, fasten loose teeth, help the falling down of uvula and ulcers in the mouth and throat. A decoction of the bark of the root is considered a specific for removal of tapeworm.
METHOD: Decoction—8 oz. of coarse bark of the root is put into a vessel and 3 pt. of cold water poured upon it. Boil for 1 hour, strain and boil it down until it measures 1 pint.
DOSAGE: Teacupful doses. Repeat if necessary, every 4 hours. For removal of tapeworm take a purgative after the first dose.

LOOSENESS OF THE BOWELS

PLANT: Life Everlasting   *Antennaria dioica*
WHERE FOUND: America, Asia, Europe
PART USED: Herb
ACTION: Astringent
USE: Taken internally as a styptic for looseness of the bowels. Also used as a gargle.

LUST, TO STOP

PLANT: Lady's Smock   *Cardamine pratensis*
WHERE FOUND: Great Britain, in low-lying places
PART USED: Herb and flowers
ACTION: Antiscorbutic, digestive, diuretic
USE: It is regarded a powerful diuretic and recommended in convulsive disorders, nervous and hysteric cases and St. Vitus Dance. An infusion assists both the veins and arteries.
METHOD: Infusion of 1 oz. in 1 pt. boiling water
DOSAGE: Taken in wineglassful doses

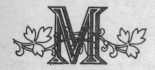

MALARIAL FEVERS

PLANT: Cashew Nut   *Anacardium occidentale*
WHERE FOUND: Native to West Indies but grows extensively in the Levant and India
PART USED: Nut, bark
ACTION: Nutritive
USE: The tree bark has proven efficient in certain malarial fevers not yielding to treatment by quinine. The nut is only edible after roasting. The fresh juice of the nut shell is acrid, poisonous and corrosive, and the West Indians use it for removing warts and corns.

MALNUTRITION

PLANT: Dog-Rose   *Rosa canina*
WHERE FOUND: Almost universal
PART USED: Whole ripe fruit (hips)
ACTION: Corrects nutritional deficiencies
USE: The hips (this applies to all rose species) if eaten as found on the shrub are almost a complete food. They contain invert sugar, citric acid and ascorbic acid (vitamin C). Excellent food for infants and children who lack proper food. Best when completely ground up "meats" and seeds are sprinkled on food or even put into babies' bottles. Also made into a syrup and a conserve.
METHOD: Use in any of its many forms; that is, whole, ground or powdered
DOSAGE: Eat as much as you like, but eat it

MENTAL EXHAUSTION

PLANT: Ginseng   *Panax quinquefolium*
WHERE FOUND: China, Eastern U.S. and Canada
PART USED: Root
ACTION: Stimulant and tonic
USE: Of value in any condition where nervous or mental exhaustion is concerned. Accepted as being beneficial in loss of appetite, stomach and digestive affections.
METHOD: Powdered Root
DOSAGE: 15 grains immediately after meals

MILK SECRETION OF NURSING MOTHERS, TO INCREASE

PLANT: Castor Oil Plant   *Ricinus communis*
WHERE FOUND: Native to India, but grown in gardens
PART USED: Leaves or oil from seeds
ACTION: Cathartic, purgative
USE: Mild acting. Especially adapted for young children and pregnant women, in cases of constipation, colic and diarrhea. Externally used for itch, ringworm and cutaneouts complaints. The nauseous taste can be disguised by orange juice or lemon juice. The Canary Island child-bearing women use the fresh leaves applied to their breasts to increase the flow of milk.
METHOD: Oil of ricinus
DOSAGE: 60 to 240 min.

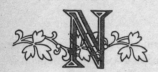

NERVE STIMULATING TONIC

PLANT: Kola — *Cola vera*
WHERE FOUND: Sierra Leone, North Ashanti, and also other tropical countries
PART USED: Seed
ACTION: Cardiac, diuretic, nerve stimulant, tonic
USE: Because of the amount of Caffeine it contains, Kola acts as a good tonic. The Africans use it and it enables them to perform arduous tasks without food. Often prescribed for alcoholism.
METHOD: Powdered kola
DOSAGE: 15 to 45 gr.

NERVES

PLANT: Basil — *Ocimum basilicum*
WHERE FOUND: Planted widely in gardens, of Asiatic origin
PART USED: Herb
ACTION: Aromatic, carminative
USE: Successfully used for centuries in mild nervous disorders. In South America it is used as a vermifuge.
METHOD: Make a hot tea—1 teaspoonful to a pot of water
DOSAGE: Drink as tea, and also added to salads and soups.

NERVOUS DEBILITY, IRRITATION AND HYSTERICAL AFFLICTIONS

PLANT: Valerian   *Valeriana officinalis*
WHERE FOUND: Europe
PART USED: Rhizome
ACTION: Anodyne, antispasmodic, nervine
USE: This herb may be used in all cases of nervous debility, irritation and hysterical affections. Also, it allays pain and promotes sleep. It is strongly nervine without any narcotic effects.
METHOD: Infusion of 1 oz. to 1 pt. of boiling water
DOSAGE: Wineglassful doses

NEURALGIA

PLANT: Lady's Slippers   *Cypripedium pubescens*
WHERE FOUND: North America, Europe and Asia
PART USED: Rhizome
ACTION: Antispasmodic, nervine, tonic
USE: Especially good for allaying neuralgic pains. Promotes sound slumber, relieves headache and female weakness. Given in hysteria and nervous disorders.
METHOD: Powdered root taken in water sweetened with honey
DOSAGE: 1 dr.

NEW ZEALAND CURE-ALL

PLANT: Kumarhou   *Pomaderris elliptica*
WHERE FOUND: North Island of New Zealand
PART USED: Herb
ACTION: Stimulant, tonic
USE: The Maoris regard it as a general cure-all, especially for blood conditions. Claimed to be beneficial in

cases of asthma, bronchitis and rheumatism. When combined with Vinca Rosea or alone, it is recommended for diabetes.

METHOD: Infusion of ½ oz. of herb to 1 pt. boiling water
DOSAGE: Wineglassful doses daily for at least 6 weeks

NOCTURNAL INCONTINENCE OF URINE

PLANT: Kava Kava   *Piper methysticum*
WHERE FOUND: South Sea Islands
PART USED: Root
ACTION: Diuretic, stimulant, tonic
USE: Used in the east to strengthen the bladder and prevent the nocturnal incontinence of urine.
METHOD: Root
DOSAGE: 1 dr.

NOSEBLEED

PLANT: Fluellin   *Linaria elatine*
WHERE FOUND: Europe and Great Britain
PART USED: Herb
ACTION: Astringent
USE: Recommended for internal bleeding, profuse menstruation and bleeding of the nose. It consolidates and strengthens.
METHOD: Infusion of 1 oz. herb to 1 pt. boiling water taken internally or applied to wounds
DOSAGE: Wineglassful as desired

OBESITY

PLANT: Samphire   *Crithmum maritimum*
WHERE FOUND: Grows along the seacoast in Europe
PART USED: Herb
ACTION: Diuretic
USE: It is reputed to be an excellent treatment for obesity
METHOD: Infusion of 1 oz. to 1 pt. boiling water
DOSAGE: Wineglassful doses taken freely

OBSTRUCTED PERSPIRATION

PLANT: Yarrow   *Achillea millefolium*
WHERE FOUND: Europe
PART USED: Herb
ACTION: Diaphoretic, stimulant, tonic
USE: Considered valuable in obstructed perspiration, the commencement of fevers, and colds. It is said to freely open the pores, and purify the blood.
METHOD: Infusion of 1 oz. of herbs to 1 pt. of boiling water
DOSAGE: Wineglassful doses, drunk warm, with a teaspoonful of Composition Essence added to each dose. Combined with Elder flowers and Peppermint, it forms a speedy cure for influenza and colds.

OBSTRUCTION OF THE LIVER

PLANT: Tamarac   *Larix americana*
WHERE FOUND: North America
PART USED: Bark
ACTION: Alternative, diuretic, laxative
USE: Highly esteemed in obstruction of the liver, jaundice, rheumatism, and skin disorders. Externally it is valuable in piles, menorrhagia, dysmenorrhea.
METHOD: Decoction of bark, mixed with spearmint, juniper, horseradish, etc.
DOSAGE: Taken in wineglassful doses

OBSTRUCTIONS OF THE GALL

PLANT: Couchgrass or Dog's Grass   *Agropyron repens*
WHERE FOUND: Everywhere (unhappily, as gardeners wail)
PART USED: Rhizome
ACTION: Aperient, demulcent, diuretic
METHOD: Infusion of 1 oz. to 1 pt. of boiling water
DOSAGE: Taken in wineglassful doses several times a day

OPHTHALMIA AND INDOLENT ULCERS

PLANT: Chickweed   *Stellaria media*
WHERE FOUND: Common weed almost everywhere
PART USED: Herb
ACTION: Demulcent, cooling
USE: The fresh leaves have long been used, with great benefit, as a poultice for indolent ulcers and ophthalmia. An ointment has been used in treatment for cutaneous diseases. For scurvy and kidney conditions an infusion has proven a good remedy.
METHOD: Infusion of 1 oz. of herb to 1 pt. boiling water
DOSAGE: Wineglassful three or four times daily

OPIATE

PLANT: Lettuce, Wild or Lettuce-opium
Lactuca virosa
WHERE FOUND: Central and Southern Europe
PART USED: Dried juice, leaves
ACTION: Anodyne, expectorant, sedative
USE: Has been used when opium cannot be given. Most frequently it is used in the form of a syrup to sooth irritable coughs when such an agent is required. Used as an anodyne.
METHOD: Lactucarium is obtained by cutting the stem in sections and collecting the latex. Lettuce-opium is usually in angular fragments or quarters, curved on one side, indicating removal from a cup or saucer in which the milky juice has been collected and dried. Externally, it is dark reddish brown, internally, opaque and wax-like. Odor, resembling opium; taste very bitter.
DOSAGE: Lactucarium—5 to 15 gr.; Syrup— 2 dr.

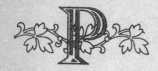

PAINS, INTERNAL AND EXTERNAL

PLANT: Cajuput   *Melaleuca leucadendron*
WHERE FOUND: East Indies
PART USED: Oil
ACTION: Antispasmodic, diaphoretic, stimulant
USE: The natives of Molucca Islands, where the tree grows, regard it very highly as a remedy for all sorts of pains, internal and external. Made into a lotion it can be used with benefit for rheumatic complaints, toothache, neuralgia, sprains and bruises. Internally taken on sugar in doses of 1 to 10 drops as a valuable diffusive stimulant in colics, spasms, flatulence and hiccough.
METHOD: Oil of cajuput
DOSAGE: 1 to 3 min.

PARASITICIDE AND INSECTICIDE

PLANT: Larkspur   *Delphinium consolida*
WHERE FOUND: European plant but naturalized wherever gardens are found
PART USED: Seeds
ACTION: Antibiotic
USE: A tincture of the seeds is effectively used as a parasiticide and insecticide. Old remedy for destroying lice and nits in the hair.
METHOD: Tincture of 1 oz. to 1 pt. dilute alcohol
DOSAGE: 10 drops and gradually increased

PAROXYSMAL ASTHMA

PLANT: Euphorbia   *Euphorbia hirta*
WHERE FOUND: Many tropical countries and India
PART USED: Herb
ACTION: Anti-asthmatic
USE: Best known and used for the prompt relief it gives
to sufferers of paroxysmal asthma.
METHOD: Infusion of 1 oz. to 1 pt. boiling water
DOSAGE: Tablespoonful doses as wanted

PELVIC FULLNESS

PLANT: Evening Primrose   *Oenothera biennis*
WHERE FOUND: America, but also grown in Europe and
Great Britain
PART USED: Leaves and bark
ACTION: Astringent and sedative
USE: Has been tested for various ailments and with con-
siderable success in the treatment of gastrointestinal
disorders of a functional origin. Proven remedy for hep-
atic torpor, dyspepsia and female disorders connected
with pelvic fullness. Of value in spasmodic asthma and
whooping cough.
METHOD: Liquid extract
DOSAGE: ½ to 1 fluid dr.

PEPPER-UPPER

PLANT: Avens or Colewort   *Geum urbanum*
WHERE FOUND: Europe
PART USED: Root
ACTION: Astringent, stomachic, styptic, tonic
USE: Claimed by some authorities to be the equal of
Peruvian Bark in action in intermittent fevers. Has a

pleasant taste. Has been used as an antiseptic remedy in cholera morbus and dysentery. Also, in weakness of the stomach.

METHOD: 1 oz. powdered root to 1 pt. boiling water

DOSAGE: Wineglassful doses three or four times a day

PESTILENT FEVERS

PLANT: Barberry, Common   *Berberis vulgaris*

WHERE FOUND: Europe

PART USED: Berries

ACTION: Diuretic, mild purgative, tonic

USE: Useful in diarrhea, dysentery, jaundice, intermittent fever and bronchitis.

PILES

PLANT: Pilewort   *Ranunculus ficaria*

WHERE FOUND: Europe and Western Asia

PART USED: Herb

ACTION: Astringent

USE: Pilewort, as its name indicates, is chiefly used for piles, for which it is almost a specific. Internally an infusion is used. Generally this is sufficient to cure most cases.

METHOD: Infusion of 1 oz. to 1 pt. boiling water

DOSAGE: Wineglassful doses

PILES AND CHRONIC CONSTIPATION

PLANT: Cascara Sagrada   *Rhamnus purshiana*

WHERE FOUND: West coast of North America

PART USED: Bark

ACTION: Laxative and tonic

USE: The bark must be more than a year old before it is

used. Largely used for habitual constipation, dyspepsia and digestive complaints, and also for piles.

METHOD: Powdered bark

DOSAGE: 20 to 40 gr. at bedtime

PLAGUE

PLANT: Sage, Garden   *Salvia officinalis*

WHERE FOUND: Southern Europe

PART USED: Leaves

ACTION: Aromatic, astringent

USE: Culpeper states: "The juice if drank with vinegar, is good for the plague. Gargles are made with sage, rosemary, honeysuckles, and plantain, boiled in wine or water, with some honey or alum added, to wash sore mouths and throats. Sage is boiled with other hot and comforting herbs, to bathe the body and the legs in the summer time, especially to warm cold joints or sinews, troubled with the palsy and cramp, and to comfort and strengthen the parts. It is recommended against the stitch, or pains in the side coming of wind, if the place be fomented warm with the decoction thereof in wine, and the herb also after boiling be laid warm thereunto."

PLAGUE AND PESTILENCE

PLANT: Juniper   *Juniperus communis*

WHERE FOUND: Widely distributed

PART USED: Berries and wood

ACTION: Carminative, diuretic, stimulant

USE: Juniper Berries were used by the ancient herbalists of Greece and Arabia and by the Romans. The juice from the berries is recommended, as commonly are many herbs, against the bitings of vipers and against the plague and pestilence.

PLAGUE, FEVER OR HORROR

PLANT: Tormentilla   *Potentilla tormentilla*
WHERE FOUND: Europe
PART USED: Root and occasionally the herb
ACTION: Astringent, tonic
USE: Parkinson writes, ". . . and so doth also the distilled water of the herbe and roote, rightly made and prepared, which is to steepe them in wine for a night and then distilled in Balneo marie; this water in this manner prepared taken with some Venice Treakle, and thereupon being presently laid to sweate, will certainly by God's help, expell any venome or poison, or the plague, or any fever or horror, or the shaking fit that happeneth . . ."

PLEURISY

PLANT: Crawley   *Corallorhiza odontorhiza*
WHERE FOUND: United States
PART USED: Rhizome (a parasitic leafless herb)
ACTION: Diaphoretic, sedative
USE: Regarded of great value for the treatment of all fevers and pleurisy. It can be relied upon to produce free perspiration.
METHOD: Infusion of 1 oz. to 1 pt. boiling water
DOSAGE: Hot small cupfuls till results are produced

POLYPUS, HEMORRHAGES AND MUCOUS DISCHARGES

PLANT: Bistort   *Polygonum bistorta*
WHERE FOUND: Europe; likes shady places
PART USED: Root
ACTION: Astringent
USE: Joseph Miller recommends the root for incontinence of urine.
METHOD: Decoction of 1 oz. to 1 pt. water
DOSAGE: Wineglassful as indicated

PREMATURE BALDNESS

PLANT: Rosemary   *Rosmarinus officinalis*
WHERE FOUND: Mediterranean regions
PART USED: Herb
ACTION: Astringent, diaphoretic, tonic
USE: Used externally, an infusion combined with borax will prevent premature baldness and also makes an excellent hair wash.
METHOD: Infusion of 1 oz. herb to 1 pt. boiling water

PROLAPSE OF THE WOMB

PLANT: Madonna Lily   *Lilium candidum*
WHERE FOUND: Native to southern Europe, but grows widely in gardens
PART USED: Bulb
ACTION: Astringent, demulcent, mucilaginous
USE: Combined with Life Root it is of value in treating prolapse of the womb and other female complaints.
METHOD: Decoction of the bulb in milk taken internally
DOSAGE: Wineglassful doses

PSORIASIS, ECZEMA AND SCROFULA

PLANT: Chaulmoogra   *Taraktogenos kurzii*
WHERE FOUND: India and Malaysia
PART USED: Seeds from which the oil is pressed
ACTION: Dermatic, sedative
USE: The oil from the seeds has been said to give good results as an internal and external remedy in scrofulous and rheumatic skin afflictions. It has also proven itself a valuable remedy in stiffness of joints and skin eruptions such as psoriasis and eczema.
METHOD: Emulsion or ointment
DOSAGE: External ointment made of 1 part of oil to 4 of base. Internal, the oil is administered in the form of an emulsion with milk or ground almonds.

PULMONARY COMPLAINTS

PLANT: Borage   *Borago officinalis*
WHERE FOUND: Throughout Europe; also grown in many gardens
PART USED: Leaves
ACTION: Demulcent, diuretic, emollient, cooling
USE: Used in France for fevers and pulmonary disorders. Externally used as a poultice for inflammatory swellings.
METHOD: Infusion of 1 oz. leaves to 1 pt. boiling water
DOSAGE: Take in wineglassful doses

PULMONARY COMPLAINTS

PLANT: Beth Root   *Trillium erectum*
WHERE FOUND: North America
PART USED: Rhizome
ACTION: Alterative, astringent, tonic, expectorant
USE: Useful in cases of internal bleeding, profuse menstruation and pulmonary complaints. Valuable in female disorders for the uterine organs. Was widely used by American Indians.
METHOD: One tablespoonful of powder in a pint of boiling water
DOSAGE: Take freely in wineglassful doses

PULMONIC CATARRH

PLANT: Pleurisy Root   *Asclepias tuberosa*
WHERE FOUND: North America
PART USED: Root
ACTION: Antispasmodic, carminative, cathartic, diaphoretic, expectorant, tonic
USE: The name clearly suggests what time has made it famous for. Its greatest use is in pleurisy, in which condition it mitigates the pain and relieves the difficulty in breathing. Of immense value in all chest complaints and

promotes a specific action on the lungs, assisting expectoration, subduing inflammation and exerting a generally mild tonic effect on the system. Highly recommended in pulmonic catarrh.

METHOD: Infusion of 1 teaspoon of the root to 1 cup of boiling water

DOSAGE: One or two cupfuls a day, cold

PUS IN BLADDER

PLANT: Corn Silk   *Zea mays*
WHERE FOUND: Wherever corn is grown
PART USED: Flower pistils of corn
ACTION: Demulcent, diuretic
USE: Recommended as a valuable remedy in various urinary problems and bladder infections. Considered especially useful in purulent decomposition of urine in the bladder.
METHOD: Infusion of 2 oz. in 1 pt. boiling water
DOSAGE: Take freely

PYORRHEA

PLANT: Witch Hazel   *Hamamelis virginiana*
WHERE FOUND: America
PART USED: Bark and leaves
ACTION: Astringent, sedative, tonic
USE: Valuable in staying internal and external hemorrhages. Useful in piles. Recommended for pyorrhea.
METHOD: For bleeding piles an ointment made by adding 1 part fluid bark extract to 9 parts simple ointment is used as a local application. For pyorrhea massage the gums daily with Liquor Hamamelides.

QUINSY AND MUMPS

PLANT: Cudweed   *Gnaphalium uliginosum*
WHERE FOUND: Common in Great Britain; grows well in most barren places
PART USED: Herb
ACTION: Astringent
USE: Regarded as an excellent remedy for quinsy.
METHOD: Infusion of 1 oz. to 1 pt. boiling water
DOSAGE: Wineglassful doses or as a gargle

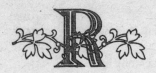

RASHES AND ITCHING

PLANT: Labrador Tea   *Ledum latifolium*
WHERE FOUND: North America
PART USED: Leaves
ACTION: Diuretic, expectorant
USE: A strong decoction has been recommended for external use as a remedy for itching. Very useful in coughs, colds, bronchial and pulmonary complaints when taken internally as an infusion.
METHOD: Internal—Infusion of 1 oz. to 1 pt. boiling water; External—Use a stronger decoction.
DOSAGE: Decoction applied to affected parts; Infusion taken in wineglassful doses

RECTAL COMPLAINTS

PLANT: Horse Chestnut   *Aesculus hippocastanum*
WHERE FOUND: Native of North Asia
PART USED: Bark and fruit (seeds)
ACTION: Astringent, narcotic, tonic, cooling
USE: The fruits have been successfully used for rectal complaints, backaches, piles, neuralgic and rheumatic disorders and hemorrhoids. The bark is used in intermittent fevers. For ulcers the bark is used in external applications.
METHOD AND DOSAGE: Bark infusion of 1 oz. to 1 pt. boiling water, taken in teaspoonful doses four times a day. Fruits: Tincture 1 in 10 of proof spirit, 10 drops morning and night.

RELAXATION OF UVULA

PLANT: Hollyhock, Common　　　　　*Althaea rosea*
WHERE FOUND: In most gardens everywhere
PART USED: Flowers
ACTION: Demulcent, diuretic, emollient
USE: Useful in chest complaints; similar action to marshmallow.

RINGWORM

PLANT: Jewel Weed　　　　　*Impatiens biflora*
WHERE FOUND: North America, East Indies
PART USED: Herb
ACTION: Aperient, diuretic
USE: An excellent application for piles is made from fresh plants boiled with lard. The juice is reputed to cure ringworm and to remove warts and corns. In jaundice and dropsy the decoction is used.
METHOD: Decoction of 1 oz. to 1 pt. boiling water
DOSAGE: Wineglassful 3 to 4 times a day

RUPTURES

PLANT: Rupturewort　　　　　*Herniaria glabra*
WHERE FOUND: England and Europe
PART USED: Herb
ACTION: Astringent, diuretic
USE: Used in catarrhal infections of the bladder.
METHOD: Infusion of 1 oz. to 1 pt. boiling water
DOSAGE: Take freely

RUPTURES AND BURSTINGS

PLANT: Five-Leaf-Grass   *Potentilla reptans*
WHERE FOUND: Common plant found widely scattered
PART USED: Herb, root
ACTION: Astringent, cooling
USE: Found useful in diarrhea and looseness of the bowels. Used externally as an astringent lotion.
METHOD: Infusion of 1 oz. herb to 1 pt. boiling water
DOSAGE: Wineglassful doses

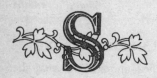

SCARLET, TYPHOID AND INTERMITTENT FEVERS

PLANT: Eucalyptus　　　　　　　　*Eucalyptus globulus*
WHERE FOUND: Native to Tasmania and Australia; cultivated in Southern Europe
PART USED: Leaves and oil distilled from them
ACTION: Antiseptic, antispasmodic, stimulant
USE: In Australia it is a household remedy for many complaints. Has potent antiseptic qualities. Used as a local application in growths and wounds. Found beneficial in ulcers. Also suggested for croup and spasmodic throat difficulties.
METHOD: Local application for ulcers, 1 oz. added to 1 pt. lukewarm water. For local injections, ½ oz. to 1 pt. lukewarm water. Internally, for scarlet fever, typhoid and intermittent fevers, the fluid extract is used and the oil is often applied freely to the body. Also used in this way for croup and spasmodic throat troubles.

SCIATIC PAINS

PLANT: Goutwort　　　　　　　　*Aegopodium podagraria*
WHERE FOUND: A troublesome weed in Europe and the British Isles
PART USED: Herb
ACTION: Diuretic, sedative
USE: Recommended internally for sciatic pains; also for

aches in joints and gout. Used externally as a fomentation.
METHOD: Liquid extract
DOSAGE: ½ to 1 dr.

SCIATICA OR ACHE IN THE HIPBONE

PLANT: Poplar   *Populus tremuloides*
WHERE FOUND: North America and Europe
ACTION: Diuretic, stimulant, tonic
USE: Universal tonic, so it is described. Said to take the place of Peruvian Bark and Quinine.
METHOD: Liquid extract
DOSAGE: 1 dr.

SEDATIVE

PLANT: Asparagus   *Asparagus officinalis*
WHERE FOUND: Europe and Asia, but now cultivated everywhere
PART USED: Root
ACTION: Cardiac, diuretic, laxative, sedative
USE: Long used because it is claimed to produce copious diuresis. It is recommended in dropsy, enlargement of the heart, and it has laxative qualities. This is the same asparagus used as the well-known food delicacy.
METHOD: Freshly squeezed juice
DOSAGE: Take in tablespoonful doses

SEDATIVE FOR THE NERVOUS SYSTEM

PLANT: Caroba   *Jacaranda caroba*
WHERE FOUND: South Africa and South America
PART USED: Leaves
ACTION: Alterative, diaphoretic, diuretic, sudorific
USE: It appears to have a sedative effect on the nervous system but is rarely prescribed.
METHOD: Liquid extract
DOSAGE: 10 to 15 gr.

SEXUAL SEDATIVE

PLANT: Pussy Willow   *Salix discolor*
WHERE FOUND: North America
PART USED: Bark, berries
ACTION: Anaphrodisiac, sexual sedative, tonic
USE: Comes highly recommended and widely used in treatment of spermatorrhea and nocturnal emissions. Relieves ovarian pain.
METHOD: Infusion of 1 oz. bark to 1 pt. boiling water
DOSAGE: Wineglassful doses

SHINGLES, ECZEMA AND SCROFULA

PLANT: Walnut, English   *Juglans regia*
WHERE FOUND: Native to Persia but grown worldwide
PART USED: Bark, leaves
ACTION: Alterative, detergent, laxative
USE: Has long been used in herpes or shingles, eczema and scrofula, taken as an infusion. Externally this is used as an application to skin eruptions and ulcers.
METHOD: Infusion of 1 oz. bark or leaves to 1 pt. boiling water
DOSAGE: Wineglassful doses as indicated

SHORTNESS OF BREATH

PLANT: Nettle   *Urtica dioica*
WHERE FOUND: Universal
PART USED: Flower, leaves, seeds
ACTION: Astringent, diuretic, nutritive, tonic
USE: The seeds are used in coughs and shortness of breath. The herb makes a pleasant nutritional beer. It is also used as a medicine in nettle rash.
METHOD: Infusion of 1 oz. of herb or seed to 1 pt. boiling water
DOSAGE: Wineglassful doses

SINGING IN THE EARS

PLANT: Savory, Summer   *Satureia hortensis*
WHERE FOUND: Garden plant grown throughout the world in gardens
PART USED: Herb
ACTION: Aromatic, carminative
USE: Culpeper says of Summer Savory, "The juice heated with a little oil of roses, and dropped into the ears, easeth them of the noises and singing in them, and of deafness also. Outwardly applied with flour, in manner of a poultice, it giveth ease to the sciatica . . ."

SKIN CLEANSER

PLANT: Lovage or Tang Kui   *Levisticum officinale*
WHERE FOUND: Southern Europe
PART USED: Root
ACTION: Aromatic, carminative, diuretic, stimulant, stomachic
USE: Used in febrile complaints, dysmenorrhea and in stomach disorders.
METHOD: Liquid extract
DOSAGE: 5 to 30 min.

SKIN CLEANSER AND IMPROVER

PLANT: Elecampane   *Inula helenium*
WHERE FOUND: Parts of Europe and Asia; grown for botanical medicine use in Europe
PART USED: Root
ACTION: Alterative, diaphoretic, diuretic, expectorant
USE: Usually mixed with other remedies for pulmonary troubles and coughs.
METHOD: Decoction of 1 oz. to 1 pt. boiling water
DOSAGE: Wineglassful doses as desired

SKIN DISEASES

PLANT: Boneset *Eupatorium perfoliatum*
WHERE FOUND: North America and Europe
PART USED: Herb
ACTION: Diaphoretic, expectorant, laxative, tonic
USE: Will be found a certain remedy in cases of fever and influenza; also for catarrh and skin diseases. When used moderately it acts rapidly and effectively.
METHOD: An infusion of 1 oz. to 1 pt. boiling water
DOSAGE: Frequent wineglassfuls, hot to induce perspiration or cold as a tonic

SORE THROAT

PLANT: Cuckoopoint *Arum maculatum*
WHERE FOUND: Europe and the British Isles
PART USED: Root
ACTION: Diaphoretic, expectorant
USE: A remedy internally and externally for sore throat.
METHOD: Powdered root
DOSAGE: 10 to 30 gr. NOTE: Large doses cause gastric inflammation and fatal results have been recorded.

SPLEEN AND LIVER COMPLAINTS

PLANT: Cup-Plant *Silphium perfoliatum*
WHERE FOUND: India
PART USED: Rhizome
ACTION: Alterative, diaphoretic, tonic
USE: Long known as a general restorative. Years have established its value in spleen and liver complaints; also useful in fevers.
METHOD: Decoction of powdered root
DOSAGE: Wineglassful doses at intervals

SPONGY AND BLEEDING GUMS

PLANT: Rhatany   *Krameria triandra*
WHERE FOUND: Bolivia and Peru
PART USED: Root
ACTION: Astringent, tonic
USE: It is useful as an application to spongy and bleeding gums. Used internally with good results in passive hemorrhages, mucous discharges and menstrual complaints.
METHOD: Extract
DOSAGE: 5 to 15 gr.

SPONGY GUMS AND SORE THROAT

PLANT: Catechu, Black   *Acacia catechu*
WHERE FOUND: India and Burma
PART USED: Extract from leaves and young shoots
ACTION: Astringent
USE: Used as a local application in relaxed sore throat and sponginess of gums. Useful for arresting excessive mucous discharges and for checking hemorrhages.
METHOD: Powdered Catechu
DOSAGE: 5 to 15 gr.

STERILITY

PLANT: Leek   *Allium porrum*
WHERE FOUND: Common garden vegetable
PART USED: Bulb, juice
ACTION: Diuretic, stimulant
USE: The Leek has long been esteemed in barrenness, as has Speedwell. Highly esteemed by the French and Germans. Constipation must be avoided.
METHOD: Expressed juice
DOSAGE: Teaspoonful doses

STIFF NECK

PLANT: Woollen or Cotton Thistle   *Carlina vulgaris*
WHERE FOUND: Mediterranean regions
PART USED: Root, leaves
ACTION: Antiscorbutic, nervine
USE: Matthew Robinson wrote in his herbal, "Dioscorides and Pliny write, that the leaves and roots taken in drink, cure stiff neck. Galen says that the roots and leaves are good for such persons that have their bodies drawn together by spasm or convulsion, or other infirmities; as the rickets in children, a disease that hinders their growth, by binding their nerves, ligaments, etc. It is good also in nervous complaints."

STIMULANT

PLANT: Buchu   *Barosma betulina*
WHERE FOUND: South Africa; especially in the Cape area
PART USED: Leaves
ACTION: Diaphoretic, diuretic, stimulant, tonic
USE: It exorts a direct effect on the urinary organs, with much benefit. Also useful in gravel, inflammation and catarrh of the bladder.
METHOD: An infusion of 1 oz. of leaves to 1 pt. boiling water
DOSAGE: Wineglassful doses three or four times a day

STIMULANT AND HEAT PRODUCER

PLANT: Cayenne   *Capsicum frutescens*
WHERE FOUND: East Indies, India, Japan, Africa and
tropical America
PART USED: Fruit
ACTION: Carminative, stimulant, tonic
USE: Considered the purest and most positive stimulant
in the herbal materia medica. May cause redness of skin.
METHOD: Capsicum powder
DOSAGE: ½ to 2 gr.

STINGS BY BEES AND WASPS

PLANT: Blue Mallow   *Malva sylvestris*
WHERE FOUND: Europe and the British Isles
PART USED: Herb, flowers
ACTION: Demulcent, mucilaginous, expectorant
USE: The infusion is a popular remedy for coughs, colds
and bronchial complaints. A fomentation is used to
soften abscesses.

Joseph Miller said, "A cataplasm of the leaves applied
to the place, stung by bees or wasps, eases the smart."
METHOD: Infusion for coughs, etc.: 1 oz. to 1 pt. boiling
water
DOSAGE: Wineglassful three times a day

STINKING BREATH

PLANT: Rest Harrow   *Ononis spinosa*
WHERE FOUND: Mediterranean areas
PART USED: Root
ACTION: Diuretic
METHOD: It is recorded that in former times the young
shoots and tender stalks before they become prickly
were pickled and eaten. Recommended against a stink-
ing breath, and to take away the smell of wine.

STONES AND GRAVEL IN THE BLADDER

PLANT: Hydrangea · · · · · · · · · · *Hydrangea arborescens*
WHERE FOUND: Native to the United States, but grown widely
PART USED: Root
ACTION: Cathartic, diuretic, nephritic
USE: Long recognized as a valuable remedy for the removal of stone and gravel in the bladder. Its best known use is in the prevention of any gravelly deposits.
METHOD: Infusion of 1 oz. root in 1 pt. boiling water
DOSAGE: Take hot or cold in wineglassful doses

STONES IN KIDNEYS AND BLADDER

PLANT: Birch, European · · · · · · · · · · *Betula alba*
WHERE FOUND: Europe, but similar tree in North America
PART USED: Bark and leaves
ACTION: Astringent, bitter
USE: Most of the old herbalists claim that the juice of the leaves when young or the water distilled from them, or the water from the tree after it has been bored with an auger, being taken for some days together, breaks the stone in the kidneys and bladder.
METHOD: Infusion of 1 oz. leaves to 1 pt. boiling water
DOSAGE: Small wineglassfuls as required

STRANGE SIGHTS AND FANCIES—
HALLUCINATIONS

PLANT: Bugle · · · · · · · · · · *Ajuga reptans*
WHERE FOUND: Throughout Europe
PART USED: Herb
ACTION: Aromatic, astringent
METHOD: Infusion of 1 oz. to 1 pt. boiling water
DOSAGE: A wineglassful taken frequently

STY

PLANT: Witch Hazel   *Hamamelis virginiana*
WHERE FOUND: Native to the United States
PART USED: Bark, leaves
ACTION: Astringent, sedative, tonic
USE: Most valuable in checking internal and external hemorrhages; also for the treatment of piles. A decoction made from the bark or leaves makes an excellent injection for bleeding piles. An ointment made by adding 1 part fluid extract bark to 9 parts simple ointment is also used as a local application. For treatment of sty in the eye, careful application of the ointment has proven effective.
METHOD: Ointment
DOSAGE: Local application

STYPTIC AND PURGATIVE

PLANT: Rhubarb   *Rheum palmatum*
   (Not Common Rhubarb which is known as Rhaponticum)
WHERE FOUND: China
PART USED: Rhizome
ACTION: Astringent, aperient, stomachic, tonic
USE: In small doses the powder will stop diarrhea; in large doses it is a simple and safe purgative. It is said to be one of the most valuable remedies that we possess.
   Externally it is used as an astringent or styptic to stop bleeding.
METHOD: Tincture or powder
DOSAGE: Sprinkle powder lightly over bleeding area

SUPPURATING TUMORS

PLANT: Onion   *Allium cepa*
WHERE FOUND: Universal
PART USED: Bulb
ACTION: Diuretic, expectorant
USE: Roasted onion as a poultice for suppurating tumors. The same treatment is used for earache. A syrup made from the juice makes a beneficial cough medicine. For gravel and dropsical afflictions onions are macerated in Gin to make a tincture.

SUPPURATION PREVENTIVE

PLANT: Marigold or Pot Marigold   *Calendula officinalis*
WHERE FOUND: Mediterranean areas; widely grown in gardens
PART USED: Petals, herb
ACTION: Diaphoretic, stimulant
USE: Generally used as a local remedy. Taken internally it assists the local action and prevents suppuration. Used for chronic ulcers and varicose veins.
METHOD: Infusion of 1 oz. of herbs and petals to 1 pt. boiling water
DOSAGE: Tablespoonful to wineglassful doses, and also as an application for external purposes

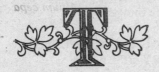

TAPEWORM

PLANT: Embelia   *Embelia ribes*
WHERE FOUND: India
PART USED: Fruit
ACTION: Carminative, diuretic, vermifuge
USE: The Indians use it in dyspepsia and rheumatic conditions. It is best known and mainly used for its ability to expel tapeworms.
METHOD: The seed (fruit) when powdered is used mixed with milk
DOSAGE: Take 1 to 3 tsps. mixed with milk, on an empty stomach, followed by a purgative

TARTAROUS INCRUSTATIONS ON THE TEETH

PLANT: Strawberry   *Fragaria vesca*
WHERE FOUND: Europe
PART USED: Fruit, leaves and root
ACTION: Astringent, diuretic, nervine
USE: They dissolve the tartarous incrustations upon the teeth. Persons afflicted with the gout or stone have found great relief by using them profusely. The bark of the root, like that of the tormentil, and the rest of its congener, is astringent. The leaves are cooling and diuretic: an infusion of them is good in the strangury; and when made strong, in the jaundice; when dried and reduced to

powder, they are astringent, and useful in fluxes of the bowels; and a strong decoction of them, sweetened with honey, is a good gargle for sore throats.

THROAT INFECTIONS, HOARSENESS, INFLAMMATORY DISEASES

PLANT: Black Currant   *Ribes nigrum*
WHERE FOUND: Grown widely in gardens; highly esteemed for jams and jellies
PART USED: Leaves, fruit
ACTION: Leaves are detergent, diuretic, cooling
USE: Very useful in febrile and inflammatory diseases, in hoarseness and infections of the throat
METHOD: Infusion of 1 oz. in 1 pint of boiling water
DOSAGE: Take in teacupful doses

THROAT RELAXER

PLANT: Oak Galls   *Quercus infectoria*
WHERE FOUND: Greece, Syria and Turkey
PART USED: The excrescence or the gall
ACTION: Astringent
USE: Used as a gargle it will smooth and relax the throat. Also used in cholera, diarrhea, dysentery and passive hemorrhages. The infusion may be used as an injection in leucorrhea
METHOD: Infusion of 1 oz. herb to 1 pt. boiling water
DOSAGE: Wineglassful, as gargle

THRUSH

PLANT: Myrrh   *Commiphora molmol*
WHERE FOUND: Arabia and North East Africa
PART USED: Oleo-gum-resin
ACTION: Healing antiseptic, stimulant, tonic
USE: A valuable and deservedly popular medicine. The

tincture is used in thrush, inflammatory sore throat, ulcers, bad legs, and other complaints. It makes an excellent wash for ulcerated mouth and tongue.
METHOD: Tincture of Myrrh
DOSAGE: 30 to 60 min.

THRUSH (LITTLE ULCERS IN THE MOUTH)

PLANT: Arsesmart   *Polygonum hydropiper*
WHERE FOUND: Europe, but naturalized everywhere
PART USED: Herb, leaves
ACTION: Diuretic, stimulant
USE: It cures those little ulcers in the mouth commonly called the thrush; and the distilled water, drunk to the quantity of a pint or more in a day, has been found serviceable in the gravel and stone. It is a diuretic of considerable efficacy, and has frequently been administered with success in the jaundice, and the beginning of dropsies. The express juice of the fresh-gathered plant appears to be the best preparation of it, and may be taken with safety to the amount of two or three ounces for a dose.
METHOD: Infusion of 1 oz. of leaves in 1 pt. of cold water
DOSAGE: Wineglassful doses as wanted

THYROID GLAND, TO IMPROVE
FUNCTION OF

PLANT: Bladderwrack   *Fucus vesiculosus*
WHERE FOUND: Off the British coasts and other coasts
PART USED: Whole plant
ACTION: Alterative, diuretic, purifying
USE: Said to have the ability to clear away obstructions by opening the natural passages of the body. Has been used for centuries as an animal food, especially during the winter. Said to keep animals in excellent health.

It was employed for making iodine of benefit for fatty degeneration of the heart, stomach and intestinal conditions, difficult breathing and dyspnea. The drug acts on the thyroid gland by furnishing iodine and thus improves its functions. Has a moldy, salty, but not unpleasant flavor.

TIRED FEET AND WEARINESS

PLANT: Lady's Bedstraw   *Galium verum*
WHERE FOUND: Europe and naturalized in North America
PART USED: Herb
ACTION: Alterative, diuretic
USE: Has been used for gravel, stone, urinary disease, epilepsy and hysteria
METHOD: Infusion of 1 oz. herb to 1 pt. boiling water
DOSAGE: Wineglassful doses several times a day

TONIC

PLANT: Peruvian Bark   *Cinchona officinlias*
WHERE FOUND: South America
PART USED: Bark
ACTION: Astringent, tonic, cooling
USE: Claimed in some respects to be one of the most remarkable remedies ever discovered. Must be properly used—not abused. For years there has been a strong tendency to overdose and this undoes the many benefits that might accrue from the use of this fine herbal remedy. Used for a tonic and nervous dyspepsia, dyspepsia due to lack of hydrochloric acid in the stomach, bowel pains due to accumulation of gas, intermittent fevers, malaria, ringing in the ears, catarrh, colds and complaints brought

on by colds, liver and spleen disfunction, jaundice, gastro-duodenal catarrh, painful periods, asthma worsened by bad weather, influenza, pains in limbs and joints, debility, nervous exhaustion, and last, but not least, it is wonderful for rebuilding the body after an exhaustive illness.

METHOD: Tincture

DOSAGE: Take 5 to 10 drops in warm water three times a day

TOOTHACHE

PLANT: Pellitory of Spain   *Anthemis pyrethrum*
WHERE FOUND: Southern Europe
PART USED: Root
ACTION: Pungent, stimulant
USE: When chewed, it excites a glowing heat, with a discharge of saliva, which relieves toothache and rheumatic complaints of the face, it is also recommended in lethargic complaints and paralyses of the tongue.

TRANQUILITY

PLANT: Asafetida or Devil's Dung   *Ferula foetida*
WHERE FOUND: Afghanistan, Persia
PART USED: Oleo-gum-resin
ACTION: Antispasmodic, expectorant, nervine, stimulant
METHOD: A pinch of the powdered gum-resin in a glass of hot water
DOSAGE: Taken hot in wineglassful doses before bedtime and before meals

TREMBLING OF THE HEART

PLANT: Dodder   *Cuscuta europaea*
WHERE FOUND: British heaths
PART USED: Herb
ACTION: Aperient, hepatic, purifying
USE: Opens the obstructions of the liver, and is good in jaundice and for the spleen.
METHOD: Decoction of 1 oz. to 1½ pts. of water
DOSAGE: Wineglassful doses as required

TREMORS OF THE LIMBS

PLANT: Lily of the Valley   *Convallaria majalis*
WHERE FOUND: Common garden flower
PART USED: Flower
ACTION: Cardiac, diuretic, stimulant, tonic
USE: An infusion of the flowers constantly taken instead of tea is an excellent remedy for nervous headaches, trembling of the limbs and other similar complaints.

TRUE TONIC, SUPER EXCELLENT

PLANT: Gentian   *Gentiana lutea*
WHERE FOUND: Mountain areas of Europe, Asia, elsewhere
PART USED: Root
ACTION: Tonic
USE: Rated and recognized as the most valuable and popular tonic medicine in the entire botanical kingdom. Bitter but without biting, it is the safest of all tonic herbs. Benefits the digestion and aids general debility, female weakness and hysteria.
METHOD: Powdered Root
DOSAGE: 10 to 30 gr.

TUMORS, ABSCESSES, GATHERINGS

PLANT: Ground Ivy   *Glechoma hederacea*
WHERE FOUND: Grows wild and is common to Europe and Britain
PART USED: Herb
ACTION: Astringent, diuretic, stimulant, tonic, expectorant
USE: Has wide use for many complaints. Has antiscorbutic qualities. Useful for indigestion and kidney diseases. When made into a poultice, mixed with yarrow and chamomile flowers, it is excellent for tumors, abscesses and gatherings.
METHOD: Infusion of 1 oz. herb to 1 pt. boiling water
DOSAGE: Wineglassful twice a day

TYPHUS FEVER AND SKIN DISEASES

PLANT: Contrayerva   *Dorstenia contrayerva*
WHERE FOUND: West Indies, Mexico, Peru
PART USED: Rhizome
ACTION: Diaphoretic, stimulant
USE: Its many excellent qualities make it an excellent remedy in typhus fever, dysentery and skin diseases.
METHOD: Infusion of 1 oz. in 1 pt. boiling water
DOSAGE: Wineglassful as needed.

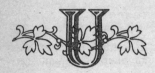

ULCEROUS WOUNDS, ASTHMA, HAY FEVER

PLANT: Comfrey   *Symphytum officinale*
WHERE FOUND: Russia, Great Britain, and transplanted anywhere
PART USED: Leaves and roots (whole plant)
USE: One of the highest rated plants in the modern herbal calendar. It appears well worth trying in any complaint that does not readily yield to other treatments.
METHOD: Used as a poultice, eaten like lettuce, or the leaves dried and made into a tea by infusion. Decoction of the root: 1 oz. of crushed root in 1 qt. of water
DOSAGE: As tea, can be drunk in cupfuls 2 or 3 times daily

ULCERS IN MOUTH AND LOOSE TEETH

PLANT: Acacia   *Acacia arabica*
WHERE FOUND: North Africa
PART USED: Bark
ACTION: Astringent
USE: It helps ulcers in the mouth and gums and fastens loose teeth.
METHOD: Bark has a high tannic acid content
DOSAGE: Use as a gargle in weak solution

ULCERS OF THE LOWER BOWELS
AND COLITIS

PLANT: Monsonia   *Monsonia ovata*
WHERE FOUND: South Africa
PART USED: Whole plant
ACTION: Aromatic, astringent
USE: It is highly recommended in South Africa for ulcerated conditions of the lower bowels. Good remedy also for acute and chronic dysentery.
METHOD: Tincture
DOSAGE: 1 to 4 dr. every three to four hours

UNIVERSAL REMEDY

PLANT: Golden Seal   *Hydrastis canadensis*
WHERE FOUND: Eastern North America; now rarely found in native, but cultivated
PART USED: Rhizome, gathered in the fall of the year
ACTION: Alterative, detergent, laxative, tonic
METHOD: Powdered Root—1 tsp. to 1 pt. boiling water
DOSAGE: 1 to 2 tsp. 4 or 5 times a day

URINARY, BLADDER AND KIDNEY
COMPLAINTS

PLANT: Broom-Corn   *Sorghum vulgare*
WHERE FOUND: United States
PART USED: Seeds
ACTION: Demulcent, diuretic
USE: Make a decoction and take it as a remedy for urinary, bladder and kidney disorders.
METHOD: 2 oz. of seeds with 1 qt. of water, boiled down to 1 pt.
DOSAGE: 1 tbs. in a glass of water at mealtimes

URINARY IRRITATION

PLANT: Arbutus, Trailing   *Epigaea repens*
WHERE FOUND: North America
PART USED: Herb (leaves)
ACTION: Astringent, diuretic
USE: This plant is reputed to be superior to Uva-ursi in all afflictions of the urinary organs attended with irritation. It is also of value in gravel and debilitated or relaxed bladder
METHOD: An infusion of 1 oz. of the leaves in 1 pt. boiling water
DOSAGE: Drink it freely

URINARY PASSAGES, INFECTIONS OF THE

PLANT: St. Johns Wort   *Hypericum perforatum*
WHERE FOUND: Europe
PART USED: Herb
ACTION: Astringent, diuretic, expectorant
USE: It is highly recommended in infections of the urinary passages.
METHOD: Infusion of 1 oz. herb to 1 pt. boiling water
DOSAGE: Wineglassful doses

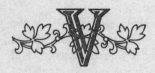

VALVULAR HEART DISEASE

PLANT: Lily of the Valley   *Convallaria majalis*
WHERE FOUND: Europe
PART USED: Flowers, leaves, whole plant
ACTION: Cardiac tonic, diuretic
USE: The syrup helps to procure rest and to settle the
brain of frantic persons, by cooling the hot temperature
of the head. The distilled water of the flowers is very
effectual and is recommended to take freckles, spots and
sunburn from the face and other parts of the body.
METHOD: Infusion of ½ oz. of the herb to 1 pt. boiling
water
DOSAGE: Tablespoonful doses

VERMIN DESTROYER

PLANT: Sabadilla   *Schoenocaulon officinale*
WHERE FOUND: Guatemala, Mexico, Venezuela
PART USED: Seeds
ACTION: Acrid, bitter
USE: It is used to destroy vermin
METHOD: Acetum (1 in 10)—Ointment (1 in 4)

VERTIGO

PLANT: Woundwort   *Stachys palustris*
WHERE FOUND: Europe
PART USED: Herb
ACTION: Antiseptic, antispasmodic
USE: An old remedy used to relieve cramp, pains in the joints, gout, falling sickness and vertigo. The bruised leaves when applied to a wound will arrest bleeding and heal the wound. The fresh juice is made into a syrup and taken internally to stop hemorrhages and dysentery.

VOMITING

PLANT: Cascarilla   *Croton eleuteria*
WHERE FOUND: Jamaica and Bahamas
PART USED: Bark
ACTION: Aromatic, stimulant, tonic
USE: Used in convalescence from acute diseases and to prevent vomiting. Also used in dyspepsia, flatulence and diarrhea. When burnt, it gives off an aromatic odor and is thus used as a fumigant.
METHOD: Infusion of 1 oz. to 1 pt. boiling water
DOSAGE: Tablespoonful to a wineglassful as required

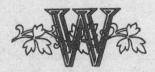

WARTS AND FUNGOID GROWTHS

PLANT: Thuja   *Thuja occidentalis*
WHERE FOUND: North America
PART USED: Leaves and tops
ACTION: Expectorant, irritant, vermifuge
USE: Recommended in chronic coughs, fever, gout, etc. Externally it is used for removal of warts and fungoid growths.
METHOD: 1 oz. of herb in 1 pt. of boiling water, taken internally
DOSAGE: Tablespoonful to wineglassful doses

WOMB DISEASE

PLANT: Dogwood or Red American Osier

                               Cornus sericea
WHERE FOUND: North America
PART USED: Bark and bark of root
ACTION: Astringent, bitter, tonic
USE: An infusion has been proven useful in checking vomiting due to pregnancy and disease of the womb. Has also been used in diarrhea, dropsy, dyspepsia and fevers.
METHOD: Infusion of 1 oz. of bark in 1 pt. boiling water
DOSAGE: Tablespoonful 4 or 5 times a day, or more

WOUNDS

PLANT: Primrose   *Primula vulgaris*
WHERE FOUND: English wild flowers
PART USED: Herb, root
ACTION: Antispasmodic, astringent, vermifuge
USE: In the early days of medicine, this plant constituted an important remedy in muscular rheumatism, paralysis and gout.
METHOD: Infusion of the root
DOSAGE: Tablespoonfuls

HERBAL COMPOUNDS

These herbal compounds from the archives of an old herbal family have been tested for over 75 years. They claim these compounds have never failed; I am inclined to be less emphatic and say that they have seldom failed.

FOR GOUT AND RHEUMATISM

Couchgrass	½ oz.
Wood Betony	½ oz.
Prickly Ash Bark	½ oz.
Sarsaparilla Root	½ oz.
Guaiacum Raspings	¼ oz.

FOR BACKACHE AND THE KIDNEYS

Pellitory of the Wall	½ oz.
Parsley Piert or Buchu	½ oz.
Broom or Wild Carrot	½ oz.
Juniper Berries	½ oz.

BRONCHITIS COMPOUND

Hyssop	½ oz.
Comfrey Root	½ oz.
Horehound	½ oz.
Coltsfoot Leaves	½ oz.
Liquorice Juice	¼ oz.

COLDS AND INFLUENZA COMPOUND

Yarrow	½ oz.
Peppermint	½ oz.
Elder Flowers	½ oz.
Chillies	½ doz.

FOR VARIOUS NERVE TROUBLES

Scullcap	½ oz.
Mistletoe	½ oz.
Wood Betony (or Vervain)	½ oz.
Peruvian Bark	¼ oz.

BLOOD PURIFYING COMPOUND

Sarsaparilla Root	½ oz.
Burdock Root	½ oz.
Sassafras Bark	½ oz.
Yellow Dock Root	½ oz.

STOMACH AND LIVER COMPOUND

Barberry Bark	½ oz.
Agrimony	½ oz.
Centaury	½ oz.
Meadowsweet	½ oz.
Ginger Root, crushed	¼ oz.

To any of the aforementioned compounds, add two pints of cold water, bring to the boil and gently simmer (with lid on) for 10 minutes. Allow to cool. The Cold and Influenza Compounds should be taken freely if the patient remains indoors.

SORE THROAT AND GARGLE COMPOUND

For all sore throats, quinsies, etc. Far safer and far better than all the antibiotics, with NO side effects.

Ragwort	½ oz.
Red Sage	½ oz.
Chillies	½ doz.

Pour over one pint of boiling water. When cold, pour off approximately half the liquid into another jug and add to this four tablespoonfuls (2 oz.) Cider Vinegar. This should be used as a gargle freely. The other half still standing on the herbs should be taken as a medicine, two tablespoonfuls three times daily.

AROMATIC

Sage	½ oz.
Rosemary	½ oz.
Thyme	½ oz.
Wild Thyme	½ oz.
Hyssop	½ oz.
Marjoram	½ oz.
Wormwood	½ oz.
Peppermint	½ oz.

Prepare as an infusion.

FOR HEADACHE

Rosemary	½ oz.
Thyme	½ oz.
Wild Thyme	½ oz.
Wild Marjoram	½ oz.
Peppermint	½ oz.
Lavender Flowers	½ oz.
Rose Flowers	½ oz.
Marjoram	½ oz.

Prepare as an infusion.

FOR CHEST AND LUNGS

Marshmallow Flowers	½ oz.
Mallow Flowers	½ oz.
Coltsfoot Flowers	½ oz.
Violet Flowers	½ oz.
Mullein Flowers	½ oz.
Red Poppy Flowers	½ oz.
Catsfoot Flowers	½ oz.

Prepare as an infusion.

TO EXPEL WORMS

Tansy	½ oz.
Wormwood	½ oz.
Wormseed (Levant)	½ oz.
Chamomile	½ oz.

Prepare as an infusion.

HEALTH TEA

Fennel	½ oz.
Cream of Tartar	½ oz.
Elder Flowers	1 oz.
Aniseed	1 oz.
Senna Leaves	2 oz.

Prepare as an infusion.

A SOOTHING COMPOUND

Marshmallow Flowers	½ oz.
Mallow Flowers	½ oz.
Mullein Flowers	½ oz.
Pellitory-of-the-Wall	½ oz.

Prepare as an infusion.

TO INCREASE THE FLOW OF URINE

Asparagus Root	½ oz.
Parsley Root	½ oz.
Celery Root	½ oz.
Fennel	½ oz.
Butcher's Broom	½ oz.

Prepare as a decoction.

TO CAUSE SWEATING

Marshmallow Root	4 oz.
Liquorice Root	2 oz.
Orris Root	2 oz.
Ground Ivy	2 oz.
Aniseed	½ oz.
Coltsfoot Leaves	2 oz.
Red Poppy Flowers	1 oz.
Mullein	1 oz.

Prepare as an infusion.

TO RESTORE NORMAL FUNCTIONS OF THE BODY

Sassafras Wood	½ oz.
Elder Flowers	½ oz.
Red Poppy Flowers	½ oz.
Borage Leaves	½ oz.

Prepare as an infusion.

TO EXPEL WIND AND EASE GRIPING PAINS

Aniseed	½ oz.
Fennel	½ oz.
Caraway	½ oz.
Coriander	½ oz.

Prepare as an infusion.

TO STIMULATE THE APPETITE

Holy Thistle	½ oz.
Germander	½ oz.
Centaury	½ oz.
Buckbean	½ oz.

Prepare as an infusion.

TO PREVENT OR STOP SPASM

Yarrow Herb	½ oz.
Orange Flowers	1 oz.
Valerian Root	1½ oz.

Prepare as an infusion.

TO COUNTERACT CATARRH

Goosefoot	½ oz.
Rupturewort	½ oz.

Prepare as an infusion.

FOR CONSTIPATION

Wormwood	½ oz.
Wood Betony	½ oz.
Bugle	½ oz.
Mountain Mint	½ oz.
Water Germander	½ oz.
Hyssop	½ oz.
Ground Ivy	½ oz.
Yarrow	½ oz.
Marjoram	½ oz.
Periwinkle	½ oz.
Rosemary	½ oz.
Sanicle	½ oz.
Sage	½ oz.

Thyme	½ oz.
Wild Thyme	½ oz.
Germander	½ oz.
Vervain	½ oz.
Arnica Flowers	½ oz.
Catsfoot Flowers	½ oz.
Coltsfoot Flowers	½ oz.

Prepare as an infusion.

FOR SEXUAL DEBILITY

Kola	1 oz.
Damiana	1 oz.
Saw Palmetto	1 oz.

Use fluid extract, 1 oz. of each, mixed together. Dosage: Small teaspoonful three times a day.

FOR HEMORRHOIDS OR PILES

Pilewort	1 oz.
Yarrow	1 oz.
Senna Pods	1 oz.
Guaiacum Chips	2 oz.
Poplar Bark	1 oz.
Raisins	2 oz.

Boil in 4 pints of water and simmer down to 1 pint. Take a tablespoonful three times a day.

FOR BLEEDING PILES

| Silver Weed | 2 oz. |
| Tormentil Root | 1 oz. |

Boil in 2 pints of water and take a tablespoonful three times a day.

FOR HIVES

Stinging Nettles	1 oz.
Yarrow	1 oz.
Golden Seal	¼ oz.
Dandelion Root	2 oz.

Simmer for 20 minutes in 2 pints of water and take a tablespoonful every four hours.

OVARIAN CYSTS

Liquorice Root	2 oz.
Yarrow	1 oz.
Comfrey	1 oz.
Yellow Dock	1 oz.
Dandelion	1 oz.

Boil in a pint of water for an hour, strain and take one tablespoonful three times daily.

NEURASTHENIA

Lady's Slipper	1 oz.
Vervain	1 oz.
Valerian	1 oz.
Scullcap	1 oz.
Saw Palmetto	1 oz.
Raspberry Leaves	1 oz.
Peruvian Bark	1 oz.
Liverwort	1 oz.
Kola Nuts	1 oz.
Barberry Bark	1 oz.
Mistletoe	1 oz.

Add 5 pints of water and simmer down to 2 pints, and add ½ oz. of Essence of Cayenne. Take one tablespoonful three times a day after meals.

FOR TOXIC CONDITION OF THE BODY

Yellow Dock   ½ oz.
Queen's Delight   ½ oz.

Make an infusion, using one pint of boiling water, and take wineglassful doses several times daily after food.

FOR HELP IN MENOPAUSE

Clivers   1 oz.
Wood Betony   1 oz.
Sanicle   1 oz.
Chamomile   1 oz.

Prepare as an infusion—1 oz. to 1 pt. of water. Take wineglassful doses after meals. Keep the bowels open.

FOR MIGRAINE

Golden Seal   1 oz.
Dandelion Root   1 oz.
American Mandrake   ½ oz.

Decoction. Take in wineglassful doses half an hour before food.

GUIDE TO
THERAPEUTIC ACTION

ALTERATIVE: Blue Flag, Burdock, Echinacea, Figwort, Mezereon, Poke Root, Queen's Delight, Red Clover, Sarsaparilla, Turkey Corn, Yellow Duck.

ANODYNE: Aconite, Coca, Henbane, Hops, Indian Hemp, Jamaica Dogwood, Poppy.

ANTIBILIOUS: Balmony, American Mandrake, Wild Yam.

ANTIPERIODIC: Alstonia, Ash, Cinchona, Feverbush, Quebracho, Wafer Ash, White Willow.

ANTISCORBUTIC: Lemon, Lime Fruit, Scurvy-Grass, Shepherd's Purse.

ANTISEPTIC: Barberry, Echinacea, Eucalyptus, Golden Seal, Southernwood, Thyme, White Pond Lily, Wild Indigo.

ANTISPASMODIC: Asafetida, Black Haw, Chamomile, Black Cohosh, Cramp Bark, Gelsemium, Lady's Slipper, Lobelia, Mistletoe, Pulsatilla, Skullcap, Stramonium, Sundew, Valerian.

APERIENT: Rhubarb, Pale Rose.

APHRODISIAC: Damiana, Muirapuama, Saw Palmetto, Yohimbe Bark.

AROMATIC: Allspice, European Angelica, Angostura, Basil, Bugle, Burnet Saxifrage, Calamus, Canella, Cinnamon, Condurango, Cubeb, Golden Rod, Magnolia, Meadowsweet, Melilot, Musk Seed, Orange, Summer Savory, Tonka Beans, Winter's Bark.

ASTRINGENT: Avens, Bayberry, Bistort, Blackberry, Catechu, Cranesbill, Nettle, Oak, Pinus Bark, Rhatany, Tormentilla, Witch Hazel.

BALSAMIC: Clary, Larch.

BITTER: Angostura, Bugle, Canchalagua, Cascara Amarga, Cedron, Chiretta, Feverfew, Gentian, Gold Thread, Horehound, American Red Osier, Quassia.

CARDIAC: Asparagus, European Birch, Butterbur, Foxglove, Hawthorn, American Hellebore, False Hellebore, Kola, Lily-of-the-Valley, Mescal Buttons, Mountain Laurel, Night-Blooming Cereus, Strophanthus, Tonka Beans, Tree of Heaven.

CARMINATIVE: Allspice, Angelica, Aniseed, Balm, Calamus, Cinnamon, Cloves, Fennel, Ginger, Peppermint.

CATHARTIC: American Black Alder, Bitter Apple, Black Root, Broom, White Bryony, Alder, Buckthorn, Butternut, Cabbage Tree, Castor Oil, Colchicum, Copaiba, Croton, Dyer's Greenweed, Gladwin, Hedge-Hyssop, Black Hellebore, Hemp, Agrimony, Holly, Hydrangea, Indian Physic, Ivy, Jalap, American Mandrake, Mountain Flax, Poke Root, Rhubarb, Senna, Squill, Swamp Milkweed, Turpeth.

CORRECTIVE: Oliver Bark.

DEMULCENT: Arrowroot, Comfrey, Couchgrass, Iceland Moss, Irish Moss, Linseed, Liquorice Root, Marshmallow, Slippery Elm.

DERMATIC: Chaulmoogra.

DETERGENT: English Adder's Tongue, Balmony, Black Currant, Goa, Golden Seal, Ragwort, Soap Tree, Soapwort, Southernwood, Walnut, Water Betony, Water Dock.

Diaphoretic and Sudorific: Angelica, Balm, Boneset, Crawley Root, Ipecacuanha, Jaborandi, Pennyroyal, Prickly Ash, Yarrow.

Digestive: Paw-Paw, Paw-Paw Seed.

Diuretic: Broom, Buchu, Clivers, Couchgrass, Hydrangea, Juniper Berries, Pareira, Parsley, Parsley Piert, Pellitory, Pipsissiwa, Shepherd's Purse, Stone Root, Uva-Ursi, Wild Carrot.

Emetic: Bitter Root, Ipecacuanha, Lobelia, Mustard, Tag Alder, Vervain.

Emollient: Linseed, Liquorice Root, Marshmallow, Slippery Elm.

Expectorant: Benzoin, Elecampane, Horehound, Ipecacuanha, Lobelia, Lungwort, Mouse-Ear, Mullein, Pleurisy Root, Polypody Root, Senega, Squill, Wild Cherry, Yerba Santa.

Cooling: Aconite, Angostura, Alstonia, Avens, Balm, Boneset, Catnip, Crawley's Root, Devil's Bit, Five-leaf Grass, Gelsemium, American Hellebore, Peruvian Bark, Wormwood.

Hemostatic: Bistort, Cranesbill, Corn Ergot, Ergot.

Hepatic: Dodder, Pichi, Yellow Toadflax.

Hydrogogue: White Bryony, American Mandrake.

Insecticide: Musk Seed, Pyrethrum.

Irritant: Bitter Apple Bryony, Cayenne, Mustard, Poison Oak, Thuja.

Laxative: Buckthorn, Cascara Sagrada, Dandelion, Golden Seal, Mandrake, Manna, Mountain Flax.

Myotic: Calabar Bean.

NERVINE: Arrach, Black Haw, Cramp Bark, Guarana, Kola, Lady's Slipper, Lime Flowers, Mistletoe, Motherwort, Muira-Puama, Oats, Pulsatilla, Skullcap, Snake Root, Sumbul, Valerian, Vervain.

NUTRITIVE: Arrowroot, Iceland Moss, Irish Moss, Salep, Saw Palmetto, Slippery Elm.

OXYTOCIC: Cotton Root.

PARASITICIDE: Cocculus indicus.

PURGATIVE: Aloes, Bitter Apple, Jalap, Mandrake, Scammony.

PURIFYING: Bladderwrack, Buckbean, Butcher's Broom, Eternal Flower, English Liverwort, Figwort, Water Dock, Wild Carrot.

RESOLVENT: Bittersweet, Galbanum.

RELIEVING CHEST CONDITIONS: Aniseed, Beth Root, Blue Mallow, Euphorbia, Hartstongue, Hyssop, Irish Moss, Jujube Berries, Labrador Tea, Life Root, Linseed, Liquorice Root, American Liverwort, Lungwort, Maiden Hair, Mullein, Polypody Root, American Sarsaparilla, Slippery Elm, Sundew, Wild Cherry.

STERNUTATORY: Asarabacca, Egyptian Soapwort Root.

STIMULANT: Ammoniac, Blood Root, Cascarilla, Cayenne, Cinnamon, Cloves, Ginger, Horseradish, Jaborandi, Kola, Mustard, Nux Vomica, Paraguay Tea, Pennyroyal, Peppermint, Peruvian Balsam, Poplar, Prickly Ash, Snake Root, Wintergreen.

STOMACHIC: Allspice, Avens, Calamus, Centaury, Chamomile, Condurango, Cubebs, Peppermint, Quassia, Rhubarb, True Unicorn Root.

STYPTIC: Avens, American Cranebill Root, Lady's Mantle.

SUDORIFIC: American Sarsaparilla, Vervain.

TONIC: Alstonia, Barberry, Bitter Root, Buckbean, Calumba, Chamomile, Chiretta, Centaury, Damiana, Gentian, Gold Thread, Hops, Kola, Nux Vomica, Peruvian Bark, Pipsissiwa, Poplar, Prickly Ash, Quassia, Strophanthus, Turkey Corn, Unicorn Root, Wild Cherry, Wormwood.

VERMIFUGE: Aloes, Butternut, Cabbage Tree, Blue Cohosh, Corsican Moss, Goat's Rue, Black Horehound, Kamala, Kousso, Male Fern, Pink Root, Primrose, Stavesacre, Tansy, Wormseed, Wormwood.

WOUND HEALING: Arnica, Crosswort, Myrrh, Water Betony.

HERBAL TEAS, TISANES, BEVERAGES AND AMBROSIALS

Contribute to the pleasantries of civilized living, aromas, fragrances, bouquets, tangs, essences, attars, pungencies and balsamics.

This flood of heavenly redolence is set free by the mere addition of hot or boiling water.

Many of these Teas have been used through the ages throughout the world for medicinal, curative, therapeutic, remedial, restorative and health-giving purposes.

ADRUE

The ground root is used for making this tea. It has a bitterish, aromatic flavor of lavender. It diffuses a feeling of warmth throughout the system and acts as a sedative.

AGRIMONY

Long used as a tea by both the English and French country folk, especially in regions where this herb is native. Agrimony used by itself makes a pleasant, enjoyable tea. Also, it is infused with licorice root and sometimes sweetened with honey, although the licorice itself is quite sweet and not much sweetening is required.

ANGELICA

It has a flavor resembling juniper berries and is used with juniper berries in making gin. Has a distinct flavor that resembles Chinese tea.

ANISE SEED

This is not generally used as a tea, but because of its sweet and unusual licorice-like taste, it is flavorful and pleasing.

BALM

Since time immemorial balm has been used as a brew to make a tasty, flavorful tea. The English flavor it with a few flowers of lavender. It is suggested that if a bit of rosemary is added, it gives the tea added character. Spearmint and cloves are also used to vary the flavor. It is very pleasant if iced and sweetening added. Has an odor and taste very similar to lemon.

BALM OF GILEAD

The buds make a balsamic tea with a pleasant odor and a slightly bitter taste.

BASIL

This is considered a gourmet tea of exquisite odor. It is also widely used to add flavor to other teas.

BAY LEAF

Has been used for centuries in both Greece and Italy as a tea. Also used to add flavor and aroma to other teas.

BEE BALM

This tea was used by the Oswego Indians and it is still used in parts of the New England states.

BARBERRY

Yes, this is the common Barberry and the berries make a pleasant acid drink of great utility.

BARLEY

Long known to be an excellent tea for the ill and ailing and for convalescents. It has much nutritional value.

BERGAMOT

A tea made from this plant was used by the American Indians and the early colonists. It is claimed that this tea has a "wild taste."

BETONY

Antonius Musa, physician to Emperor Augustus, held Betony in such high repute he wrote a long treatise devoted to this tea. Culpeper concluded that since the Emperor did not keep fools about him, Betony surely must be a worthy tea. If a bit of dried orange peel or a clove is added, it becomes even more delicious.

BILBERRY

Also known as Whortleberry. The leaves of this plant, when dried in the shade, make a tea that in flavor cannot be distinguished from Chinese tea. When the tea is made of the dried or fresh fruits, it has been proven particularly useful as a tonic.

BIRCH BARK

Another of the many teas used by the North American Indians. Our pioneers learned about these fine teas from them. The leaves of the birch are also used for making tea, as well as a combination of both bark and leaves. The brew exudes a sweet odor. Generally a most agreeable tea.

BONESET

Long recognized as a tea of bitter flavor. In the good old days among the early settlers, who lived under adverse conditions in log cabins with earthen floors where it was cold, damp and miserable, they found this Boneset tea invigorating and warming and the tea was generally used as a nightcap.

BURNET

Tea made from this herb, with lemon and sweetening added, was used by the French and the Indians.

CALAMINT

This has an aromatic, palatable, mint-like flavor, with a pleasant odor.

CARDAMOM
Makes a warm, grateful aromatic tea. It is made from the crushed fruits.

CASSIA PODS
This tea makes a pleasant fruit laxative.

CATNIP
In Britain this was long popular before they ever heard of Chinese tea.

CHAMOMILE FLOWERS
Known throughout the world and long accepted as one of the most popular teas found anywhere. It is still widely used and is served throughout Europe. Loved by the Germans and the French alike. Some people drink it just as it is. Others add a bit of ginger or include a dash of fennel or a bit of honey and a slice of lemon.

CINNAMON
Has a most unusual fragrance and is widely used in the Arab countries for its ability to refresh. It is a fragrant cordial.

COMFREY
Has a sweetish taste but no odor. Improved by adding lemon. Widely accepted as a nutrient tea. Found useful and recommended for many ailments.

CORN SILK
A mild, odorless tea with a sweet flavor. A bit of licorice or ginger adds zest.

COSTMARY
Properly it is *Chrysanthemum balsamita*, but it is also known as Mint Geranium. The leaves have a lavender-like odor to them. Makes a very flavorful, minty tea. Use it carefully. Otherwise, it is apt to get too strong. The flavor is most unusual but delightful.

CUP MOSS

Makes a most invigorating and enjoyable tea if sweetened with honey. Recommended as a beverage for children.

DAMIANA

This old fragrant tea, which dates back to the days of the Spanish conquistadors, comes to us from Mexico with the highest praise. Provides a sparkling, golden brew with a most delightful aroma and an agreeable, bitterish taste. Said to encourage pleasant, amorous dreams.

DANDELION

A tea is made from the leaves of dandelions, using 1 teaspoon to a cup. It is useful in gall bladder and rheumatic conditions.

DICTAMNUS

The flowers and foliage of this plant give off a gas which has a strong odor and will actually ignite if a lighted match is put to it on a windless summer evening. It is referred to as Limonella by the Italians, due to the strong lemon-like scent of the leaves and the seed pods. Has a most unusual flavor that is not liked by everyone.

DILL SEEDS

A tea made from dill seeds is regarded as an effective help in the case of hiccoughs. Dill seeds combined with anise seeds, chamomile and hop shoots are said to have sedative effects.

DITTANY

The leaves of this plant are dotted with aromatic oil glands. It is a native American plant which produces a most desirable tea. The pleasing aroma given off by this herb resembles a mixture of thyme and bay leaf. Exquisite.

DOG-ROSE

The fruits of the Dog-Rose, when ground up, make a sweetish and acidulous tisane. Actually, it is a good brew to give to children when it is sweetened with honey. Of course it is loaded with beneficial ascorbic acid or Vitamin C.

DWARF ELDER

The fruit of this plant makes a pleasing and invigorating tea. It is an old English favorite. With a dash of peppermint added and taken hot before retiring, it makes an excellent nightcap.

ELDER FLOWERS

Tastes sweetish at the start and then has a muscatel flavor with a touch of bitterness. Has a slight odor, but characteristic. With Peppermint added, it has long been used as a remedy against influenza.

FENNEL SEED

An agreeable tea recommended for children and the aged, when slightly sweetened with honey.

FIG

The dried figs can be soaked overnight and when hot water is added, they make a sweet, pleasing drink. It is both laxative and nutritive, and generally found to be satisfying.

FLAX SEED

Take an ounce of whole flax seed, an ounce of honey, half an ounce of licorice root and the juice of lemon. Over this pour a quart of boiling water and allow it to stand, while keeping it warm, for about four hours. Then strain off the liquor and you'll find it gratifying and palatable.

FENUGREEK

This tea has long been used by all those who are interested in health. In fact, many people prefer it to all other teas. It is frequently used to expel phlegm. The taste and flavor remind one of celery and lovage.

GALANGAL

If mixed with alfalfa and strawberry leaves, it blends into a delectable brew. It is said to have been used by the Tartars.

GINGER

This is a genuine old-time favorite. Used as a stimulant and pepper-upper for chills caused by dampness or cold weather. In the West Indies it is used with a few cloves or a dash of nutmeg. The dried and sugared ginger, cut into slivers, is frequently used.

GOLDENROD

Often referred to as Blue Mountain Tea. This tea has a faint perfume. It has long been used in Pennsylvania where it was actually considered an article of commerce. When brewed it makes a delicious golden brew and has a warm anise-like flavor and fragrance.

GRINDELIA

A tea made from the herb of this plant was very largely employed in the treatment of asthmatic and bronchial conditions, as well as in whooping cough and kidney diseases. It is a resinous plant with a strong scent. Has a decidedly medicinal flavor.

GROUND IVY

Most often it is used with a few leaves of Melissa or Lemon Verbena, Sage, Lavender Flowers or Rosemary, with a little lemon added. It can be sweetened with honey. Licorice also improves its flavor. When using licorice, honey is not required for the licorice is sweet enough. This tea requires very little steeping.

HAWTHORN

This well known plant, whose berries ripen in September, has been long used in botanic medicine, mainly for heart conditions, and it is considered most effective and helpful. The leaves are used in Germany where it is said to be more pleasing than Chinese green tea. Black Currant leaves, Balm and Sage are mixed with the Hawthorn leaves to make a most likeable brew.

HOP

Has a bitter taste and an aromatic flavor and odor. It is chiefly used as a bitter and is believed to improve appetite and digestion. It is usually taken warm upon retiring, as it is known to help induce sleep.

HOREHOUND

This herb has a most agreeable flavor and makes a refreshing, appetizing and healthful beverage. It is from this plant that they make the horehound ale. A nip of cayenne pepper, a dash of vinegar sweetened with honey, added to horehound tea, makes a most stimulating tea that is usually drunk hot at bedtime.

HORSEMINT

This tea is a good stimulant and like all of the mint family, it is serviceable and stimulating in various conditions. It makes a palatable beverage and it is also known to be a good diuretic. The taste and odor resemble that of garden mint.

HORSETAIL

Flavored with peppermint and licorice, it is exquisite and delightful.

HYDRANGEA

This plant is known in Japan and Korea and the leaves of this shrub are widely used as tea. The Japanese refer to it as *Ama-Tsja,* which in Japanese means "Tea of Heaven." The plant is widely known in cultivation in this country.

HYSSOP

A decoction of Hyssop made with figs, water, honey and rue helps the old cough.

JUNIPER

A tea made of this plant is widely used in Bohemia.

LABRADOR

This tea has been long known to the Indians of North America, especially the Chippewas. The leaves of this plant are used to make the tea and it is claimed to be soothing, fragrant and gratifying in spite of its bitter, aromatic taste with a camphor-like odor. Has been widely used for coughs, colds, bronchial and pulmonary infections. The tea is rose-colored.

LADY'S MANTLE

Use one to two teaspoons of Lady's Mantle per cup of boiling water. Allow to steep for ten minutes.

LANTANA

It is a semi-tropical North American plant, with interesting multicolored flowers. The tea is widely used but mainly by the natives where the shrub is found. It has a strong flavor and odor and is not popular, execept among the natives.

LAVENDER

Has a strong, fragrant odor that is quite characteristic of the plant. It is not often used as a tea in itself because of its rather strong flavor. It is generally mixed with other herbs. The tea is usually made from the flowers.

LEMON GRASS

This is the plant with the lemon-scented foliage. Cultivated in India for centuries. The tea made from this plant is esteemed mainly by the people of the West Indies, where it has long been regarded as a delectable brew. It is best served piping hot.

LEMON VERBENA

To obtain the highest pleasure from the drinking of regular Chinese tea, add a few leaves of Lemon Verbena. If you like it sweet, add a teaspoon of honey. When the leaves of this plant are rubbed they give off a distinct lemon-like odor and the taste resembles that of lemon.

LICORICE

The best tea is made from the ground pieces of root, not the woody sticks. The plants yield a substance known as glycyrrhiza, which is said to be fifty times sweeter than cane sugar. It is a great thirst quencher. May be used either hot or cold. It is used by itself and also with other teas.

LIME FRUIT

The juice of this fruit taken as is or with honey makes a most enjoyable tea. Often used with alcoholic beverages. One of the earliest known antiscorbutics.

LINDEN

The tea has a bouquet similar to that of Sweet Jasmine. Best served with lemon, if iced. If taken before retiring, hot, it induces pleasant sleep and is most relaxing.

LIPPIA

It has an agreeable aromatic taste and odor. Recognized as an excellent remedy for coughs, colds, whooping cough and bronchial infection.

LOVAGE

A tisane made from lovage tastes actually more like a broth than a tea. It is one of the few teas that can be drunk or taken with salt, if preferred, instead of sugar or honey. It is claimed to have the effect of an internal bath and thus acts as a deodorant.

MARJORAM

The tea is made from the herbs and leaves. It has an aromatic and agreeable flavor. Regarded as a tonic and a stimulant.

MUGWORT

Still used as a common tea in Cornwall. Sometimes mint or pennyroyal is added, and sweetened with honey. It should not be steeped very long. It is recommended for old people because of its mildness.

MULBERRY

The fruit of the Mulberry, when squeezed and the juice extracted, forms a grateful drink for convalescents and is said to check the thirst and cool the blood.

NETTLE

The herb makes a nice botanic beer. It is also used as a medicine in nettle rash. The infusion of 1 oz. either herb or seed to 1 pt. of boiling water is taken in wine-glassful doses. It is made like Chinese tea, sweetened and flavored with lemon to taste. It is also often mixed with Chinese Tea: 1 part nettles to 3 parts tea.

OLD ENGLISH

Take Hawthorn leaves, dried, 2 parts; Sage and Balm, 2 parts. Mix these well together and they will make an excellent and pleasant tea, particularly wholesome for people who must avoid stimulating beverages.

PARAGUAY

It is commonly known as Yerba or Yerba Mate. To South Americans, Yerba is the only drink. It is also widely used in North America. It definitely has stimulating properties, without the harmful effects of tea or coffee. It is used as a green leaf tea, and there is also a tea made from the bark and the stems and the leaves, all ground up into a powder. Most South Americans prefer this powder and they like it strong.

PARSLEY

A highly nutritious tea. It is often mixed with Alfalfa, yellow dock root and watercress.

PEACH

The leaves of the Peach tree are used by the Chinese in making a tea, which they claim has many medicinal uses; specifically for irritation and congestion of the gastric surfaces, as well as coughs, whooping cough and chronic bronchitis. It is taken in small quantities.

PENNYROYAL

A stimulating beverage. The taste and odor are distinctly minty, but it still retains its own characteristics. It is sometimes mixed with Lavender flowers. Most frequently taken hot upon retiring.

PEPPERMINT

Next to Chinese tea Peppermint tea is one of the most widely used of all herb teas. It deservedly earns the high esteem in which it is held. It can be given freely to children. Peppermint tea also forms the basis of many other herb teas. It is often mixed with alfalfa, clover flowers, linden flowers, chamomile, licorice, strawberry leaves, raspberry leaves and others.

PERSIMMON

The leaves of the Persimmon make a most exquisite tea. Claimed to be better than Chinese tea and is rich in Vitamin C.

PIPSISSEWA

Another one of the many Indian teas that was used by the early fur traders and pioneers. Gives off a most delightful reddish color with a rich flavor, but it is definitely bitterish. Honey or licorice will sweeten it.

POMEGRANATE

The fruit and the rind can be used in making tea. This is one of the oldest known fruits on earth.

POTENTILLA

From this plant is made a popular tea known as Five Finger Tea. It is used mainly by the folks living in the Ozarks, Arkansas, Kentucky and Tennessee. The plant is a sprawling wayside weed which resembles wild Strawberry.

PRUNE

The juice of the prune makes a most delightful and refreshing tea, and it is also a safe, sure laxative. The dried fruit is soaked for 24 to 48 hours in water and the resulting juice may then be drunk cold or hot.

QUINCE

The fruit of the Quince tree can be made into a most inviting, delicious tea. The taste, aroma and odor are entirely distinctive. Use with honey or licorice.

RASPBERRY LEAF

Used for centuries in Europe and considered especially useful for pregnant women. Widely esteemed and used. Found in many of the herbal tea blends.

RED CLOVER FLOWERS

More widely used than most people realize. Has a mild, delicate flavor. Sweeten with honey. Try it with some Chamomile flowers, too. Serve it hot or cold.

ROSEMARY

Was used many hundreds of years ago by the Arabian physicians, who were probably the first to recommend this fragrant herb as a tea. If Lavender flowers, a bit of lemon and honey are added, it becomes most inviting and captivating.

SAGE

Care must be taken not to make the brew too strong. Heavenly if sweetened with maple syrup. Sometimes flavored with a dash of orange or lemon, or a pinch of mace or cinnamon. It is also exquisite mixed with Melissa. It is claimed that the Chinese preferred Sage Tea to their own native tea and would trade twice the quantity of their choicest tea for it.

ST. JOHN'S BREAD

The pods of this plant, when ground up, make a sweet, chocolate-flavored brew. It is considered highly nutritive and is claimed to improve the voice. It requires no sweetening as the pods themselves are quite sweet.

SARSAPARILLA

Use 1 part Sarsaparilla, 1 part Sassafras, ½ part Snakeroot, and allow the tea to brew for at least five minutes. Keep the lid on the pot. Maple syrup is ideal for sweetening.

SASSAFRAS

The bark of the root ground to a powder is generally used for this tea. Only a quarter of a teaspoonful is required to make a cup. The leaves can also be used. It has definite stimulating qualities.

SENNA

It has a sweet but sickly flavor. The odor is distinctly tea-like. It is generally combined with other aromatic and stimulating herbs to modify its griping effects. But it has been used successfully for centuries as a laxative and a cathartic. Here is a suggested infusion: Senna leaves 2 oz., Ginger 1 dr., boiling water 1 pt. Let it stand for an hour, strain through muslin and take in wineglassful doses.

SLIPPERY ELM

Ground Slippery Elm bark, when boiled and strained and then flavored with lemon juice and honey, not only makes a delicious tea but something that is most nutritious, palatable and refreshing. Considered an excellent food or beverage for invalids or children.

SLOE BERRY

The young, tender leaves afford the best substitute for the foreign teas. The berries are exceptionally sweet.

SPEARMINT

Similar in its flavor and properties to Peppermint. Slightly milder and more fragrant. Useful as a beverage for children.

SPEEDWELL

Has a bitter astringent taste, with a slight fragrance. Used in Europe as a substitute for Chinese tea and thought by some to be equal or superior to it.

SUMACH BERRIES

The Ojibway Indians used the berries of this plant to make a cooling drink for summer and they boiled it hot for the winter. It has a pleasant acid flavor.

SUMMER SAVORY

It has an aromatic piquancy and taste, recalling thyme and marjoram, but distinctive. Said to be one of the most stimulating of herb teas.

SWEET BAY

In the Everglades the Seminoles use the leaves of this plant for making a tea which they highly prize as a wholesome beverage.

SWEET CICELY

Has a sweet anise-like taste or flavor. Used as a tonic and stimulant tea and is also useful in coughs and flatulence.

TEA TREE

The crew of Captain Cook's ship, as well as other early navigators, used the leaves of this tree for making tea. It is still used in New Zealand and Australia. Usually found only in the Far East.

TEA

No list of teas would be complete without listing what the world recognizes as TRUE tea, which is also known as *Thea chinesis* and *Camellia theifera*. It is an evergreen shrub that grows in the hills of China, India, Ceylon and other parts of the world. The leaf buds, together with two or three young leaves, are collected and allowed to wither. They are then rolled and fermented, and the color changes from green to black. Part of the tannin is oxidized and traces of volatile oil are produced. Green tea is obtained by drying over a fire and in this way the tannin is not oxidized and the leaves retain their green color. The principal constituents are caffeine and tannin.

146

THYME

Brew this the same way as you would Chinese tea. This brew gives off its best flavor when iced and served with lemon. Makes an excellent brew along with alfalfa, strawberry, red clover, raspberry, sassafras, licorice and others. Said to be a warming tea for the aged.

VALERIAN

Has a sweetish, bitter taste and a characteristic odor. Taken in wineglassful doses it allays pain and promotes sleep. It is of benefit to the nerves without any narcotic effects.

VERBASCUM

It is valuable when hoarse or when losing one's voice, particularly for those who speak or sing, or when having difficulty in breathing. It can be used for children and old people as well.

VERVAIN

This tea is a sedative and stimulates the production of bile. Used in nervous exhaustion and as a sedative and digestive. It is slightly bitter and soothing. Use one teaspoon of Vervain per cup. Allow to steep for only five minutes. It is said to clear the eyes and the sight.

WILD MARJORAM

Wild Marjoram tea has a flavor that resembles a blend of thyme, rosemary and sage.

WINTERGREEN

This tea is rose-colored and possesses its own natural sweet flavor. No sweetening agent need be added. The tea is unusual in that it leaves a most pleasant lingering after-taste. Said to be a very valuable remedy in the treatment of rheumatism. Of benefit to infants who have trouble with their stomachs.

WOODRUFF

By simply steeping the dried leaves to the desired strength, you will find a most fragrant and palatable brew. The herb acquires a vanilla-like aroma when it is dried. Said to be one of the most agreeable and delightful of all herb teas. Used to flavor candies, wine and liquors.

YARROW

Distinctly used as a medicinal brew by the old herbal practitioners. Used as a beverage by Swiss mountaineers. It has an insipid flavor and a feeble odor. However, combined with elder flowers, peppermint and honey, it makes an agreeable, delectable brew. Said to be of value for influenza and colds.

27/10/74 USING HERBAL TEAS

The merits of teas in herbalism are many. If they did nothing else but make it possible to avoid the use of black tea, coffee and other beverages that are made from burnt or highly heated and treated substances, they would contribute greatly to the health of the population. It is an established fact that all burnt substances are carcinogenic.

Black teas are subjected to high heat and fermentation as well as other treatments. Thus, the use of herbal teas will eliminate the dangers in that direction. Apart from this, herb teas in variety would prevent the accumulation of various components as well as the resulting deficiencies that create an imbalance in the human body.

Actually, tea is an infusion of an herb in hot water. In many cases the nutrients or food values contained within the herb are found in the resulting tea. Therefore, instead of suffering ill or harm from regular tea and other burnt substances like coffee, one would receive benefits from drinking herb tea.

It is suggested that when tea is brewed it be drunk immediately or within a few minutes after brewing. Leaving it brew, stew or sit for a long time does not enhance its pleasantness or nutritional value. However, there are some exceptions to this rule.

Where milk or sweetening is desired, by all means use it; but to obtain the best flavor and pleasure from tea, it is best without either.

Among the other benefits of herb teas are flavor, aroma, bouquet, nutrients and healing qualities.

It is not suggested that any or all herb teas are necessarily suited for drinking after or with meals, or as a daily routine.

Admittedly, serving the proper tea at the right time and knowing how to prepare it is in itself an art worth acquiring.

The method generally given is to use one teaspoonful of tea per cup and then another teaspoonful for the pot. My experience with herb teas does not indicate this rule to be valid. There are many teas where one teaspoonful per cup would be much too much. For example, with sassafras, licorice or sage, a teaspoonful per cup would be overpowering. Therefore, I would suggest that with every different brew you try different strengths and then decide the amount to be used in each case.

It is generally suggested that boiling water be used, but I have learned that you can use water hot, without being boiled, and get results that are even better. Furthermore, in this way you do not harm most of the nutrients found in the herbs.

I would set five minutes as the maximum for the steeping and then pour.

Good spring or well water is best. Try to avoid chlorinated, fluorinated or otherwise chemically treated water.

You cannot get good results from water that contains added chemicals.

The preferred pot is of course an earthenware pot. Porcelain pots are used and so are enamel pots. I consider them fair.

Do not use herb teas that have to be filtered through a sack. That is, don't use herb teas in paper or cloth bags. You will never get the true bouquet or aroma or flavor from them.

GATHER YOUR OWN HERBS

In this day and age in America the gathering and drying of herbs has become a lost art, although at no time did it ever reach the perfection that it achieved in Asia and Europe.

Nature has, in this country, as well as in all others, provided, in the herbs of its own growth, the remedies for the several diseases to which it is most subject; and although the addition of what is brought from abroad should not be supposed superfluous, there is no occasion that it should cause the other to be neglected.

The descriptions in this work very readily distinguish what are the real plants that should be used.

The virtues of different plants reside principally in certain parts of them, and those differ according to the nature of the herb. These several parts are to be selected, and the rest left. Some to be used fresh, just gathered; others, either by necessity, or by natural preference, make it proper to dry and preserve them.

In some only the leaves are to be used; in others, the whole plant cut from the root; in others, the flowers only; in others the fruits; in others, the seeds; in some, the roots; of some trees, the barks; some, the woods; and only the excrescences of others; some vegetables are to be used entire, whether fresh gathered, or dried and preserved. Of all these, instances have been given in the preceding pages, and are specified under each article, as the part of the plant to be used is named; whether fresh, or necessarily dried or preserved.

Most plants native to our country die off in winter, except the root. When the whole plant dies, the root is seldom of any value; but when the root remains many years, and sends up new shoots in the spring, it frequently has great value. This may be a general rule: there is very little to be expected in the roots of annual plants; their seeds, for the most part, contain their greatest virtues.

In others, the root lives through the winter, and there arise from it large leaves in the spring, before the stalk appears. These are to be distinguished from those which afterwards grow on the stalk, for they are more juicy, and for many purposes much better. In the same manner, some plants, from their seeds dropped in the fall, produce a root and leaves which stand all the winter, and the stalk does not rise till the succeeding spring. These are of the nature of those leaves, which rise from the root of other plants before the stalks in spring; and are in the same manner to be distinguished from those which grow upon the stalks. They have the full nourishment from the root, whereas the others are starved by the growth of the stalk and its branches, and the preparations made by nature for the flowers and seeds.

When the leaves of any plant are said to be the part fittest for use, they are not to be taken from the stalk, but these large ones growing from the root are to be chosen; and these where there is no stalk, if possible; for then only are they fullest of juice, and have their complete value.

When the juice of the leaves of any plant is required, these are the leaves from which it is to be pressed. When they are ordered in decoction, notice is always taken whether they be best fresh or dried. If fresh, they should be just gathered for the occasion. They should be cut close to the root, and shaken clean, not washed. They are to be cut into the pot. If they are to be dried, the same caution is to be used; they are best dried by spreading them upon the floor with the windows open, turning them often. When thoroughly dried, they should be put in a drawer, pressing them close, and covered with paper. When the entire plant is to be used except the root, care is to be taken that it is gathered at the proper season. Nature, in the growth of plants, tends to the production of their flowers and seeds, but when they are ripe, the rest begins to decay, having done its duty; so the time when the entire plant is in its most full perfection is when it is in bud: when the heads are formed for flowering, but not a single flower has yet blossomed—this is the exact time.

When herbs are to be used fresh, it is best to cut off the tops: three or four inches long, if for infusion, and if for other purposes, less. If they are to be beaten with sugar, they should be only an inch, or less, just as far as they are fresh and tender. The tops of the plant thus gathered are always preferable to the whole part for immediate use.

When the entire herb is to be dried, the season for gathering is to be when the flowers are budding; and the time of the day must be when the morning dew is dried away. If they are cut wet with the dew, herbs will not dry well, and if they are cut at noon, when the sun has made the leaves flag, they will not have their full power.

Care must also be taken to cut them in a dry day, for the rain will do as much harm as that of dew.

When the herbs are gathered, they are to be looked over, the decayed leaves to be picked off, and the dead ends of the stalks cut away. They are then to be tied in small bunches (the smaller the better) and the hung upon lines drawn across a room where the wndows and doors are kept open in good weather. The bunches should be half a foot apart, and they are to hang till perfectly dry. They are then taken down gently, without shaking off the buds of the flowers, and laid evenly in a drawer, pressing them down, and covering them with paper. They

153

are now ready for infusions and decoctions, and are better for distillation than when fresh.

The flowers of plants are principally used fresh, though several particular kinds retain their value when well dried. They are on these different occasions to be treated differently.

Lavender flowers, and those of stoecha, keep very well; they should therefore be preserved dry. The lavender flowers are stripped off the stalks, husk and all together, and spread upon the floor to dry. The stoecha flowers are to be preserved in the whole head. This is to be cut off from the top of the stalk, and dried in the same manner. When dry, they are kept as the herbs.

When rosemary flowers are dried, they are generally taken with some of the leaves about them, for the leaves retain more value than the flowers. Rose buds are to be dried, and to this purpose, their white heads are to be cut off. The full-blown flowers may be preserved in the same manner. The red rose is always meant, when we speak of the dried flowers.

For the rest of the flowers used in medicine, they are best fresh; but as they remain only a small part of the year in that state, the method is to preserve them in the form of syrups and conserves, such as the syrup of cloves and poppies, the conserves of cowslips, and the like.

Among the fruits of plants, several are to be used fresh, as the hip for conserve, and the quince, mulberry, and black currant, from the juices of which, syrups are made. As to those which are to be dried, as the juniper berries, the bayberries, and the like, they are only to be gathered when just ripening, not when quite mellow, and spread upon a table or floor, often turning them till they are dry.

With respect to seeds and plants, these are all to be used dry. Nature has in manner dried them to our hands for they are not to be gathered till perfectly ripe, and then they need very little additional care. They are only to be spread for three or four days upon a clean floor, where the air has free passage, but where the sun does not come. They are then ready to be put up.

The seeds used in medicine are of three general kinds. They either grow in naked heads or umbels, as in fennel, parsley, and the like; or in pods, as in mustard and cresses; or in large fleshy fruits, as in melon and cucumbers. In each case they must be left upon the plant till perfectly ripe; then they are only to be shaken from the heads upon the floor, or if in pods, a smart stroke or two of the plant upon the floor when they are thoroughly ripe will dislodge them. In the other case, the fruit must be cut open, and they must be taken out from among the wet matter, separated from the membranes that are about them, and spread upon a table, in a dry place, where they must be often turned and rubbed as they dry, that in the end they should be perfectly dry and clean.

Among the roots, a great many are to be used fresh, but a greater number are best dried. The black and white briony, the arum, and some others, lose all their value in drying; and many that retain some, yet lose the greater part of it. There are others which are excellent, both fresh and dried, as the marshmallow and some more.

The best season for gathering roots for drying, is in the early part of the spring. What nature does for plants when they are just going to flower, she does for roots when the leaves are just going to bud: the juices are rich, fresh, and full, and the value is strongest in them at this season.

At the end of February and in the beginning of March, the ground should be searched for the first budding of leaves, and the roots taken up. They are to be wiped clean, not washed, and, according to their natures, prepared for drying.

Some are full of mucilaginous juice, as marshmallow and the squill: these must be cut into thin slices crosswise, and they will dry best if laid upon a cheesecloth stretched across a frame. They must be frequently turned and be very thoroughly dry before they are put up, or they will become moldy. Rightly prepared, they keep very well.

Other roots have juices that evaporate more easily. These should be split open lengthwise, first cutting off the head, and the little end; or if considerably thick, they may be quartered. When this is done, they are strung upon a line, by drawing a needle, threaded with a small twine, through their thickest part, and they are then hung up to dry in the manner of the herbs. The line is stretched across a room, and the doors and windows should be kept open in good weather.

When roots consist of a sort of thick rind, or fleshy substance within the rind, and a hard sticky part in the middle, this fleshy substance under it possesses all the value; the hard inner substance having none. In this case, the root is to be split longwise as before, and the hard woody part is to be taken out and thrown away. The rest is to be strung, as described above, and dried in the same manner.

When roots consist of fibers, these are generally connected to a head, and the best method is to split this in two, and then string up the separate parts for drying.

As to the excrescences, such as galls of the oak, and the burr from the wild briar, they are naturally so dry, that they only require to be exposed to the air, on a table, for a few days, and they will keep a long time.

Lastly, the funguses, such as Jew's-ears, and the like, are to be gathered when they are full grown, and strung upon a line. They must dry leisurely, or else they spoil. They must be very well dried before they are up, or they will grow moldy in damp weather.

METHODS OF PREPARING

Juices are to be squeezed from leaves or roots, and in order to do this, they are to be first beaten in a mortar. There is no form whatever in which herbs have so much effect.

Juices are to be obtained in some plants from the entire herb, as in watercresses, brooklime, and others that have juicy stalks; in others the leaves are to be used, as in nettles, and the like, where the stalk is dry, and yields nothing, but is troublesome in the preparation. When the juice of a root is to be had, it must be fresh and thoroughly beaten. A marble mortar and wooden pestle serve best for this purpose, for anything of metal is improper: many plants would take a tincture from it, and the juice would be so impregnated with it as to become a different medication.

When the thick juice, fresh drawn, is too coarse for the person's stomach, it may be allowed to settle and grow clear. A little sugar may be added also in beating the herb, and in many cases, as in those juices given for the scurvy, the juice of an orange may be added, which will greatly improve the flavor.

To the roots it is often proper to add a little white wine in the bruising. The same addition may be made to some of the colder herbs. And if a little sugar, and, upon occasion, a few grains of powdered ginger, is added, there will be little fear of the medicine disagreeing with the stomach, and its effects will be the same as if it had been bruised and pressed alone.

INDEX OF
COMMON NAMES

INDEX OF COMMON NAMES

INDEX OF
BOTANICAL NAMES

INDEX OF BOTANICAL NAMES

167

Daphne mezereum, 32
Delphinium consolida, 80
Digitalis purpurea, 35
Dorstenia contrayerva, 109

Embelia ribes, 103
Ephedra sinica, 58
Epigaea repens, 112
Equisetum arvense, 42
Erythraea centaurium, 47
Eucalyptus globulus, 92
Euonymus atropurpureus, 41
Eupatorium perfoliatum, 96
Euphorbia hirta, 81
Euphrasia officinalis, 51

Ferula foetida, 107
Ferula galbaniflua, 37
Fragaria vesca, 103
Fraxinus ornus, 40
Fucus vesiculosus, 105
Fumaria officinalis, 25

Galium verum, 106
Gentiana lutea, 108
Geum urbanum, 81
Glechoma hederacea, 109
Glycyrrhiza glabra, 46
Gnaphalium uliginosum, 88
Gratiola officinalis, 50
Guaiacum officinale, 39
Guarea rusbyi, 34

Halymenia edulis, 39
Halymenia palmata, 39
Hamamelis virginiana, 87, 101
Hedera helix, 55
Helianthemum canadense, 30
Helianthus annuus, 34

Hordeum distichon, 41
Hydrangea aborescens, 100
Hydrastis canadensis, 111
Hypericum perforatum, 112

Ilex paraguensis, 49
Impatiens biflora, 90
Inula helenium, 95

Jacaranda caroba, 93
Juglans cinerea, 64
Juglans regia, 94
Juniperus communis, 83

Kalmia latifolia, 39
Krameria triandra, 97

Lactuca virosa, 79
Larix americana, 78
Laurus nobilis, 31
Ledum latifolium, 89
Leptandra virginica, 38
Levisticum officinale, 95
Lilium candidum, 85
Linaria elatine, 76
Linaria vulgaris, 45

Macrocystis pyrifera, 55
Malva sylvestris, 99
Medicago sativa, 28
Melaleuca leucadendron, 80
Melissa officinalis, 52
Mentha piperita, 62
Mentha viridis, 59
Monsonia ovata, 111
Myrica cerifera, 34
Myrrhis odorata, 27

Nepeta cataria, 30
Nymphaea odorata, 69

Ocimum basilicum, 74
Oenothera biennis, 81
Olea europaea, 31
Ononis spinosa, 99

Paeonia officinalis, 50
Panax quinquefolium, 73
Petasites vulgaris, 29
Peumus boldus, 59
Phytolacca decandra, 55
Pilocarpus microphyllus, 44
Pinus mugo, 67
Pinus sylvestris, 67
Piper methysticum, 76
Piper nigrum, 40
Plantago major, 32
Plantago psyllium, 64
Polemonium reptans, 63
Polygonum bistorta, 84
Polygonum hydropiper, 105
Polymnia uvedalia, 68
Polyporus fomentarius, 63
Pomaderris elliptica, 75
Populus candicans, 36
Populus tremuloides, 93
Potentilla anserina, 53
Potentilla reptans, 91
Potentilla tormentilla, 84
Primula vulgaris, 116
Prunella vulgaris, 64
Prunus persica, 54
Punica granatum, 70

Quercus infectoria, 104

Ranunculus ficaria, 82
Rhamnus purshiana, 82
Rheum palmatum, 101
Rhus toxicodendron, 28
Ribes nigrum, 104
Ricinus communis, 73

Rosa canina, 72
Rosmarinus officinalis, 85
Rubus villosis, 44
Rumex acetosa, 43
Rumex aquaticus, 57
Ruscus aculeatus, 65

Salix alba, 35
Salix discolor, 94
Salvia officinalis, 83
Salvia sclarea, 51
Sanicula europaea, 36
Satureia hortensis, 95
Schoenocaulon officinale,
113
Scolopendrium vulgare, 69
Scutellaria laterifolia, 60
Senecio maritimus, 35
Serenoa serrulata, 29
Sesamum indicum, 36
Silphium perfoliatum, 96
Simaba cedron, 27
Sisymbrium officinale, 60
Sorghum vulgare, 111
Spiraea ulmaria, 37
Stachys betonica, 45
Stachys palustris, 114
Stellaria media, 78
Symphytum officinale, 110

Tamarindus indica, 52
Taraktogenos kurzii, 85
Taraxacum officinale, 68
Thuja occidentalis, 115
Thymus serpyllum, 67
Trigonella foenum-
graecum, 58
Trillium erectum, 86
Turnera diffusa, 28
Tussilago farfara, 41

INDEX OF
AILMENTS AND USES

INDEX OF AILMENTS AND USES